Contents

Mentoring in Nursing
A Dynamic and Collaborative Process

Second Edition

Sheila C. Grossman, PhD, APRN-BC, FNP

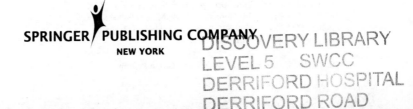

SPRINGER PUBLISHING COMPANY
NEW YORK

Springer Publishing Company, LLC
11 West 42nd Street
New York, NY 10036
www.springerpub.com

Acquisitions Editor: Allan Graubard
Composition: diacriTech

ISBN: 978-0-8261-0768-8
E-book ISBN: 978-0-8261-0769-5

12 13 14 15/ 5 4 3 2 1

The author and the publisher of this work have made every effort to use sources believed to be reliable to provide information that is accurate and compatible with the standards generally accepted at the time of publication. Because medical science is continually advancing, our knowledge base continues to expand. Therefore, as new information becomes available, changes in procedures become necessary. We recommend that the reader always consult current research, specific institutional policies, and current drug references before performing any clinical procedure or administering any drug. The author and publisher shall not be liable for any special, consequential, or exemplary damages resulting, in whole or in part, from the readers' use of, or reliance on, the information contained in this book. The publisher has no responsibility for the persistence or accuracy of URLs for external or third-party Internet websites referred to in this publication and does not guarantee that any content on such websites is, or will remain, accurate or appropriate.

Library of Congress Cataloging-in-Publication Data

Grossman, Sheila.
  Mentoring in nursing : a dynamic and collaborative process / Sheila C. Grossman. – 2nd ed.
    p. ; cm.
  Includes bibliographical references and index.
  ISBN 978-0-8261-0768-8 – ISBN 978-0-8261-0769-5 (E-book)
  I. Title.
  [DNLM: 1. Mentors. 2. Nursing. 3. Interpersonal Relations. WY 18]

  610.73–dc23

                                                        2012018596

Special discounts on bulk quantities of our books are available to corporations, professional associations, pharmaceutical companies, health care organizations, and other qualifying groups.
If you are interested in a custom book, including chapters from more than one of our titles, we can provide that service as well.

For details, please contact:
Special Sales Department, Springer Publishing Company, LLC
11 West 42nd Street, 15th Floor, New York, NY 10036-8002
Phone: 877-687-7476 or 212-431-4370; Fax: 212-941-7842
Email: sales@springerpub.com

Printed in the United States of America by Gasch Printing.

Mentoring in Nursing

Second Edition

Sheila C. Grossman, PhD, APRN-BC, FNP, received her baccalaureate and doctoral degrees from the University of Connecticut, her master's degree in biophysiological nursing with a clinical nurse specialty in respiratory nursing from the University of Massachusetts, and her post-master's certificate as a family nurse practitioner from Fairfield University. She currently is a professor and coordinator of the Family Nurse Practitioner Program at Fairfield University, Fairfield, CT, and works as a nurse practitioner weekly at an urban primary care center in Hartford.

She has presented at multiple international, national, and regional conferences as a keynote and plenary speaker on mentoring and leadership and consulted for several health care agencies. She has received grants for her research and also for program development at Fairfield University School of Nursing. Dr. Grossman received an *American Journal of Nursing Book of the Year Award* (2007) for the first edition of this book, *Mentoring in Nursing: A Dynamic and Collaborative Process*, and has other journal publications in the areas of mentoring and leadership. Currently she serves as an expert resource for the American Nurses Association on the Mentoring Project with five state nurse associations selected for mentoring grants. She also received an *American Journal of Nursing Book Award* (2009) for the third edition of *The New Leadership Challenge: Creating a Preferred Future for Nursing.* She co-authored *How to Run Your Nurse Practitioner Business: A Guide for Success* and two gerontology certification books for APRNs and RNs.

Dr. Grossman has completed the Cincinnati Children's Hospital Genetics Fellowship and the AACN Leadership Fellowship. She has practiced as a staff and charge nurse on a variety of medical–surgical and critical care units and has been a critical care instructor at Hartford Hospital, Mount Sinai, Hartford, CT, and St. Francis Hospital and Medical Center in Hartford, CT.

Dr. Grossman has received awards for innovative teaching/mentoring contributions, most recently the National Organization of Nurse Practitioner Faculty Annual Nurse Practitioner Educator Award (2011), and the Connecticut Nurses Association's Josephine Dolan Award for Outstanding Contributions to Nursing Education (2009) for demonstrated excellence in mentoring others.

She is a board member of the American Nurses Credentialing Center Commission on Certification, 2011–2015, and serves as a program evaluator for the Commission on Collegiate Nursing Education. She is an active member of the American Association of Critical-Care Nurses, the Sigma Theta Tau International Mu Chi Chapter, the National Organization of Nurse Practitioner Faculty, the Academy of Nurse Practitioners, and the American Nurses Association, and a past member of the Connecticut State Board of Nursing.

Foreword

Over the years I have mentored many individuals such as students, new nurses, experienced nurses trying something new, and faculty. At first, it seemed like a lot of work to mentor someone, but over time, mentoring strategies became easier to implement and a routine component to most interactions. In my position as dean, I am constantly reminded how much mentoring new faculty need to develop into fully contributing, robust faculty. Over the years, it has become essential to provide professional development and mentoring in order to recruit and retain new talent. Formal and informal mentoring has increased faculty performance, has increased retention and commitment to the university, and has resulted in knowledge sharing. Recently, I had the good fortune to talk with Sheila Grossman and to be introduced to this book. She is passionate about how mentoring can empower those of us in the nursing profession. Her intent is to tell us how to create a mentoring spirit in nursing.

Everyone who picks up this book can benefit from the simple and straightforward way that the content is presented. Perhaps you have questioned if you are qualified to be a mentor. Maybe you don't know how to begin. This book provides guidelines and offers strategies, so that you can begin engaging in mentoring activities right away. Your own life experiences in learning and working with others qualify you to be a mentor, so there is no question about your suitability. Your enthusiasm for your work and the profession will be so contagious that you will inspire others just by doing what you enjoy most.

Even though mentoring has long been recognized as beneficial to the development of students, practicing nurses, and faculty, there has been a lack of an established mentoring history in nursing. Yet the literature is replete with evidence about the benefits of mentoring programs or other types of programs to enculturate new graduates and new staff into an organization. You only have to imagine being a beginning student or staff member with little experience in providing care to patients in a rehabilitation setting to underscore the value of a culture of mentoring. It is obvious that strategies that increase confidence and competence and increase retention are beneficial for individuals and organizations. Advantages associated with mentoring programs are experienced by mentors as well as mentees. Benefits include pride in facilitating the professional growth of another nurse and the creation of nurses who will become mentors. Drivers of a successful experience include well-defined goals and objectives, training, evaluation, administrative support, and recognition and celebration. A well-organized mentoring program can be an effective tool to attract and retain nurses in our rapidly changing health care environment. Consequently, health care organizations are beginning to contribute substantial resources to formal mentorship programs. In order to ensure their success, it is important that mentoring programs be based on sound principles and expose participants to core mentoring skills.

This book will help you to understand how mentoring relationships are established and enable you to identify some of their key features, so that you can create effective mentoring experiences. According to Grossman, effective mentoring relationships have clearly identifiable stages or phases that reflect their growth and progress, so you will be able to analyze your experiences. You learn how to become more proactive by taking part in mentoring within the nursing profession to promote successful leadership and professional development.

You've done yourself a favor by picking up this book. It will soon become obvious that every professional nurse can excel as a mentor, preceptor, and coach. Give mentoring a try and see where you end up. Enjoy the journey.

Janet M. Brown, PhD, RN
Dean and Professor
Valparaiso University
College of Nursing
Valparaiso, IN

Preface

The intent of this book is to help nurses, educators, administrators, and nursing students change the ways nurses do things, frequently separate from others and always in the same lock-step structured manner. It promotes empowerment by advocating for, and developing, the mentoring spirit in nursing as conducive to the best possible health work environment where reciprocal encouragement, recognition, and respect are predominant themes.

Nurses who feel that little is right at their work settings, who are interested in developing their leadership abilities and empowering themselves and others, and who are interested in obtaining recognition for their work, their unit or department, agency, professional organization, or institution should read this book. Anyone interested in joining the mentoring culture of nursing, and who feels she or he can encourage others and has the potential to change the health care setting into a high-performance, healthy, caring work environment, will benefit from this book.

The second edition of *Mentoring in Nursing: A Dynamic and Collaborative Process* provides multiple perspectives on the process of mentoring and how nurses can do great things for themselves and their profession through mentoring. The literature base for the book includes a broad range of multidisciplinary resources focused on outcomes. Certainly, mentoring can assist people in being better than what they would be solely by themselves. Once a mentee becomes self-empowered, there is a greater likelihood of being more creative, better able to adjust to changes, to be visionary, to manage conflict effectively, to take risks, to communicate effectively, and to be a critical thinker. It is evident that the closeness that develops between mentors and mentees sparks energy and creativity that assist individuals in maximizing their talents. Precepting and coaching are also discussed as subareas of mentoring.

Generally, nurses seem to use the word *mentorship* interchangeably with the preceptorship and coaching relationship. Mentoring seems to be perceived as an all-encompassing term for many nurses and the term *mentor* often refers to anyone helping or guiding another individual in his or her job or career. This book uses the term *mentorship* as the process of mentoring, which can include precepting and coaching and also defines multiple types of mentorships.

Chapter 1 describes the process and evolution of mentoring with short descriptions of precepting and coaching; types, components, and stages of the mentoring process; a rationale for each relationship; characteristics of classic mentoring; advantages and disadvantages of mentoring; and how the additional support roles of the preceptor or coach might influence mentoring. Chapter 2 relates how nurses have begun to develop a mentoring culture, best practices regarding mentoring in nursing, culturally competent mentoring, and some examples of mentoring in nursing. Chapter 3 discusses the concept of empowerment; strategies to help empower oneself, others, and the profession; a comparison of empowerment with the enabling process; and how healthy work environments for nurses impact a mentoring culture. Chapter 4 analyzes characteristics of effective mentors, mentees, and mentoring. It stresses that one size, or type, of mentoring program does not necessarily fit all needs. The generational gap of nurses and how this influences a mentoring culture are discussed along with strategies to assist with mentor-mentee pairing. Chapter 5 describes methods for capturing the role of an effective mentor; delineates characteristics of effective mentors, preceptors, and coaches; and identifies benefits for those who participate in some form of mentoring. Chapter 6 discusses effective mentee relationships, ideas for choosing an effective mentor or mentors, suggestions for maximizing one's potential for being chosen by an effective mentor, and both the benefits and possible negatives of being in a mentoring relationship. Chapter 7 presents the need for more outcome measurement in mentoring, suggests some variables to evaluate which measurements impact mentoring, and gives some examples of mentoring outcomes. Chapter 8 summarizes the advantages of early mentoring, suggests incentives for mentors and mentees, and discusses the implications of what a mentoring culture will do for the profession of nursing, the organizations that employ nurses, and the mentors and mentees themselves.

Everyone has a part to play in a mentoring relationship, and it is a myth that only older and more experienced individuals can be mentors. Isn't it true that any form of energy can mentor or inspire us? How many times have you encountered this energy? Have you perhaps missed some of these stimulating exchanges? Have you become so entrenched in your own agenda that you have lost contact with the network and have eventually found yourself outside the network? So many talented people have been marginalized in their organizations due to the "out-networked phenomenon." How does one get back on track?

Mentoring in Nursing was written to assist nurses in identifying how anyone who wants to, and is willing to, can be re-networked into a successful mentoring relationship or relationships. Mentoring in nursing encompasses a reciprocal guided experience, whether it be formally or informally assigned over a mutually agreed-on period of time, that empowers the mentor and mentee to develop personally and professionally within a caring, collaborative, culturally competent, nonevaluated, and respectful environment.

The professional aspect is especially important because it needs to include not just what the mentoring can do for the mentee and the mentor but also what it can do for the nursing profession. Essentially, the profession must foster a mentoring culture that offers networking to all who want to take advantage of it and are willing to give to it. Probably one of the best ways to get on track is to be part of a team that partners with other effective teams or groups interested in similar outcomes, continually work on developing your leadership skills, and encourage others whom you interact with to do the same.

The major points in this book revolve around several themes:

- The importance of being more flexible in working with others and changing how we currently do certain things
- The need to empower oneself to be a leader in order to make a difference
- Creating a mentoring spirit in nursing in which nurses are recognized for their expertise
- Using mentoring, precepting, or coaching in the appropriate setting and relationship

Mentoring is not a commodity that comes in a one-size-fits-all mentality; it must be individualized to each nurse according to his or her needs. The classic mentoring dyad has evolved to include multiple mentors and peer mentoring groups. Networking and partnering are imperative for organizational, professional, and individual success.

The profession stands to benefit greatly from the effects of a mentoring spirit in nursing. My hope is that nurses will be more satisfied with their work, fewer nurses will leave the profession, more nurses will enter, and fewer nurses will work in ways that can be destructive to young and new members of the profession. *Mentoring in Nursing: A Dynamic and Collaborative Process* is designed to help nurses in practice, administration, and educational roles understand the benefits of mentoring others as well as the value of being mentored themselves.

Acknowledgments

This book is dedicated to the multiple nurses who mentor, precept, and coach other nurses simply because it is the right thing to do. Ultimately a successful nurse mentor will find herself or himself in a setting that advocates for each nurse just as one tries to advocate for each patient. Did anyone ever tell you "Wow, you are like a magnet, everyone comes to you for advice and encouragement. Don't you ever get sick of helping others?" Well, you already know that if you are one of these magnets, the more you mentor others the more improvements will generally come your way. That is because, as you know, there is something in it for the mentor after all!

Great appreciation goes to the Helene Fuld Foundation, which supported my original mentoring research that greatly assisted me in writing the first edition of this book, and to Fairfield University for providing me a venue to establish a mentoring culture.

My gratitude is also extended to Janet M. Brown, PhD, RN, Dean and Professor, Valparaiso University, an excellent role model and a truly legendary mentor in nursing, for her wise and creative reflections in the Foreword of this book. Also, much thanks and appreciation go to Allan Graubard, Executive Editor, and Christina Ferraro, former Assistant Editor, at Springer Publishing Company, for their assistance in publishing this book.

I thank my many colleagues and friends who have mentored me over the years, my husband Bob, and our daughters Lisa and Beth, who have been mentors to each other and always supported me in everything I do. This book is a testament to my parents, John and Janice Carey, who were excellent role models and always allowed me the gift of time to create new ideas. I also salute my sister, Ellen C. Bernstein, who has consistently been a leading mentor in my life.

Acknowledgments

1

Mentoring: The Evolvement of a Network of Mentors, Preceptors, and Coaches

Mentoring is an encompassing term that has existed for years in many disciplines. It is also often confused with precepting and coaching. Although there have been various definitions of the term, the general purpose of mentoring has been similar in its many usages and is frequently described as a relationship between an experienced and less experienced individual that applies both to the professional and personal aspects of one's life. Certainly mentoring is not a new phenomenon, and it will undoubtedly continue to evolve from a one-to-one relationship to a more collaborative process. The term, mentoring, has become a buzzword that is used over a wide continuum, from asking for "Ned Flanders type" volunteers to mentor prison inmates in Kansas all the way to precise pairings of senior research academicians with junior faculty just starting on their research trajectories. In fact, there are mentoring workshops, such as the *Learning Across Disciplines Mentoring Workshop* recently held at the University of New Mexico Mentoring Institute (2011), that focus on multidisciplinary sharing of innovative mentoring models. There are also mentoring and coaching journals. *The National Post* (2007) describes coaching, though not mentoring, as the second fastest growing profession in the world. For its part, precepting seems to be more focused to the nursing profession.

A decade ago, McWeeny (2002) recognized an expansive concept of the mentoring process, likening it to a changing mosaic that will be more diverse and enduring. In today's world, it seems only sensible that mentoring will continue to evolve from a one-on-one relationship to a network with an overarching focus on team effort. The question remains, however, if the common base of any mentoring relationship will continue to be the classic dyad of one mentor and one mentee, or will mentoring be the term that describes any relationship where people assist each other with career transitioning and gaining new knowledge, experience, and skills. For example, the teacher role can be, and is, much more than lecturing, correcting papers and tests, and giving constructive feedback to a group of students. Rather, the relationship can evolve into a one-on-one connection that the teacher and some or all students develop over a semester. Ultimately—if both the teacher and student have some special connection—the relationship will progress into a classic one-to-one dyad mentorship or perhaps the relationship will foster rich coaching sessions within that one semester and then stop.

Many view mentoring as any process that helps another learn (Cottrell, 2006; Dungy, 2010; Maxwell, 2008; Shea & Gianotti, 2009; Zachary, 2009). This is why precepting and coaching are commonly linked with mentoring. Although the three terms are different, each describes a relationship between people. For example, *mentoring* (usually no payment is involved) can involve the classic dyad of mentor and mentee or the mentoring network that includes multiple individuals mentoring each other in various areas. *Precepting* is based on the apprentice–master framework, where a person who is newly hired is assigned to an experienced employee to learn the "job" over a prescribed amount of time (commonly 4 weeks). This relationship has no payment attached to it; rather, the preceptor is expected to orient or precept the new employee as part of their job responsibilities. *Coaching* generally depicts one person, the coach, who coaches or "supports and teaches" a group of people to accomplish a goal. Or, there is a process (generally involving payment to the coach) where the coach coaches one person in a specific area and over a predetermined amount of time to gain a skill, expand one's portfolio, or achieve a specific executive status.

This chapter thus describes the process and evolution of mentoring; provides brief descriptions of precepting and coaching and how these support roles might influence mentoring; depicts types, components, and stages of mentoring; presents a rationale for mentoring; the characteristics of classic mentoring; and advantages and disadvantages of mentoring. Of course, the lack of consensus over the definition of a relationship between two or more people to assist and support inexperienced individuals makes it difficult to compare research outcomes, especially when studies use the terms (mentoring, precepting, and coaching) interchangeably. Reviewing descriptions of mentoring, precepting, and coaching from disciplines outside nursing will help to increase our knowledge here, including about how mentoring has developed. Clarifying the differences between mentoring, precepting, and coaching will assist us in validating how mentoring has evolved as the premier collaborative relationship.

THE PROCESS OF MENTORING

Most of the research that has been published on mentoring
nursing profession is in the fields of business and education, therefore,
this chapter presents concepts that have come from studies in non-
nursing disciplines (Cottrell, 2006; Daloz, 1999; Gay, 1994; Jonson, 2008;
Kram, 1983, 1986; Levinson, Darrow, Klein, Levinson, & McKee, 1978;
Luna & Cullen, 2000; Maxwell, 2008; Murray, 2001; Ragins & Kram,
2007; Roberts, 2000; Schweibert, 2000; Shea & Gianotti, 2009; Sinetar,
1998; Stoddard & Tamasy, 2009; Zachary, 2005, 2009). Here, the term
mentoring is thought to be an offspring of human living, teaching and
learning, our giving and receiving wisdom in all relationships, in leadership, and through succession.

Although some feel a mentorship involves just two people, others
feel it can be a group of people helping each other. This perspective
reinforces the more contemporary idea that it is generally more worthwhile to reach out to, network with, encourage, and mentor others than
to work solo. However, although many people recommend a mentorship, there are always a few successful individuals who routinely work
on their own. They manage each heartache and organizational burden
alone just as they also receive merit and fame for their accomplishments alone. Even leaders generally want mentors (or at least friends
with the mentor's spirit) because they are "reaching into the unknown
for self-expression" and can use some encouragement (Sinetar, 1998,
p. 39). Can't everyone use some encouragement? Isn't success sweeter
when it is a result of a team effort?

Thus, why not extend the classic dyadic mentoring definition to
include collaborating within a larger group of people with the purpose
of creating a mentoring spirit in work groups? The following example
will clarify: Sara, a new graduate from a BSN program, begins her
new RN position on the Telemetry Unit and is immediately assigned
to Joellen to precept. Joellen, a 10-year veteran of the Telemetry Unit
and neighboring Coronary Care Unit, is the charge nurse on most
shifts she works due to her experience and Clinical Level IV status.
Sara is actually Joellen's niece and has been mentored by Joellen for
the last 4 years, since Sara began her BSN program. Joellen ensures
that the schedule has them paired on each shift, precepts Sara every
shift, and mentors her further outside of the hospital but does not tell
anyone they are related. The staff also welcomes her as a fast learner
and "good nurse." They want her to be part of their team. Sara soars in
her orientation and is acclaimed for her clinical decision-making skills,
given her brief clinical experience. Sara becomes a Clinical Level II

nurse in a short 6 months. The nurse manager wonders why Sara has performed so well when two other new RN hires are still grappling with any unstable patient. These RNs have been passed from preceptor to preceptor without anyone assuming accountability for their learning and experiences. In fact, after 6 months, both of these RNs lack confidence and are fearful of many types of patients and situations.

Essentially, these two new RN graduates were assigned a preceptor for every shift and probably accomplished all of the skills they were supposed to during orientation but never had anyone take time to help them assimilate the new skills, review the decisions an RN makes when caring for an unstable cardiac patient, or had an opportunity to develop a trusting relationship with any of the staff nurses. They were missing the "mentoring" aspect of the preceptorship. In contrast, Sara had 24/7 mentoring and precepting by the same individual and a welcoming from the staff. Due to Joellen's status on the unit, all of the staff encouraged Sara and developed good rapport with her. Sara was part of a mentoring culture while the other two RNs were still working on becoming members of the staff and trying to demonstrate they had what it takes to be telemetry nurses. Wouldn't it be ideal if each and every new staff member was welcomed, mentored, and precepted like Sara? By the way, Sara and Joellen went on to have a classic mentoring dyad relationship.

Today's work settings demands of its workers that they produce outcomes that are measurable, cost-effective, ethical, and make a difference. It stands to reason that these demands would be more easily reached if workers teamed up with each other and shared their various strengths to generate more productivity. However, it may not be as easy as it sounds. One has to imagine or, in some cases, remember, how challenging it is to motivate others, which can be difficult, extremely difficult, or sometimes simply impossible. The other side to the notion of a collaborative mentoring network is self-interest. Isn't it true that most people do not give unless they are going to receive something in return; something tangible for themselves? In this light, it is important to reflect on how mentoring evolved and came to be what it is today: a process of facilitating one's colleagues as well as one's own success.

Historically, most have thought the term, *mentoring*, was derived from *The Odyssey* where the Greek poet, Homer (1946), wrote about the wise mentor who protected the king's son in his absence. Andrews and Wallis (1999) refer to another source, *Les Aventures de Telemaque*, by Fenelon (1699/1994), when identifying the origin of the modern mentor. Although our consideration of modern mentoring has evolved appreciably, the mentor can still act in support of the mentee by protecting her or him, for example, from difficult nurses who, purposefully or by accident, can damage their colleagues; the variable "sharks" in the profession or organization. Who hasn't known a shark in the nursing profession? How many times have nurses been accused of not assisting the new and young nurses entering the profession?

Contemporary literature such as *The Lion King* with Zazu, *Karate Kid* with Daniel, and *Star Wars* with Yoda also reflect mentor and mentee characters and portray stories we can all relate to in our pasts. Equally so, each of these relationships involved more than pedagogy, as in teaching a skill or preparing someone for a position. It involved a caring and genuine fondness or friendship between mentor and mentee. Of course, it is also important that ethical principles are followed when determining who would best mentor whom and which mentee would benefit the most from whom (Sommers-Flanagan & Sommers-Flanagan, 2007).

People enjoy hearing about how someone has succeeded and tend to be proud of how their influence, no matter how small, may have helped in this effort. Zachary (2009), in her work at Leadership Development Services, identified that Gen-Xers and Gen-Yers crave mentoring by way of several attitudes: what they derive from being mentored and connected is what makes the difference in whether they are chosen for a promotion or not, and being mentored and connected is what helps them gain the courage to make that innovative change they have always dreamed about. The truth of this is exemplified in the nursing profession, in which many of today's successful nurse leaders have their educational roots in a diploma or associate degree program but have progressed through doctoral studies. Many times, their promotions have been a direct result of the connections made in their academics; connections that have allowed them to move up their career ladder in service or higher education settings. It seems that these connections among nurses and other health care providers, begun in the early stages of one's profession, are what make certain individuals more successful than others.

In 2001, with over 30 years of work behind her, Murray developed the *Facilitated Mentoring Model*, which defines *mentoring* as a process of assigning a more skilled with a less skilled person with one clear goal: increasing the mentee's skill set. Being skill focused, this almost sounds like precepting. However, the model has evolved to reflect that learning and growth, not just skill development, occur with these individuals. Murray goes on to discuss concepts such as total quality, self-managed work teams, and facilitated mentoring, and asks people in business to be more open to networking with others—with the idea that a team is more successful than an individual. Using these quality improvement methods can foster new ways of mentoring, such as networking with high performers as outside consultants, finding out new ideas from interacting with peers from one's professional organizations, and hiring a specific consulting group or individual (coaches) to come in and teach an identified needed skill. Strike and Nickerson (2011) recommended using specific *How to Mentor Modules*, illustrating what has worked previously in certain circumstances with a mentor–mentee relationship, along with consulting with one's mentor, as the tools to assist all in achieving their goals. Strike and Nickerson also felt that the mentee may at times need to ask others, either connected via the mentor's or via the mentee's own network, to help them acquire new skills or knowledge.

So how is one to expand her or his mentor network so that he or she can connect with more than one mentor for assistance? Many of those in the workforce today seek out multiple employment opportunities—either working two part-time positions, being self-employed and having multiple clients, or working one full-time position along with consulting. Working for more than one employer over a period of time seems to be more productive in a majority of fields than having one long-term employer for the majority of a career. Many believe that in order to advance one's careers, they need to have multiple employers but not necessarily at the same time. Today, most employees do not possess the same kind of loyalty that their predecessors felt, and are equally or more focused on their careers within the context of accomplishing their organization's goals. They expect to advance their careers by working in a variety of work settings, which can also facilitate the added benefit of a much broader network of mentors.

Maxwell (2008) says if one wants to grow one must be intentional about it—either working to accomplish annual goals independently or perhaps having a mentor to assist one in accomplishing such goals. Shea and Gianotti (2009) describe mentoring as a process by which one individual strives to enhance the mentee's special strengths by working closely with the person. In fact, they believe the effective mentor serves as "a tutor, counselor, friend, and foil who enables the mentee to sharpen skills and practice critical thinking" (p. 13). And mentoring constitutes more than being a product of the "good ole boy circle." Simon and Eby (2003) define mentoring as a relationship that allows junior members of a group opportunities to receive guidance, advice, and "opportunities for personal and professional development" (p. 1083). The mentor too will reap career rewards from participating in the mentoring. The potential opportunities gained from networking through a successful mentorship appear to be key for professional career growth. Although this "good ole boy" concept is present in the nursing profession, it is not accurate to think it is the only reason someone succeeds. It seems that having the right mentor who might be in the right circle of successful leaders who mentors extremely well is most beneficial for mentee success. So what is success? It can include a variety of achievements such as

- certification in one's area of specialty
- being promoted
- obtaining a new, higher level position at another organization
- receiving grant funding
- achieving a top administrative position in one's work field or academia
- election to lead a national or international organization
- appointment to a prestigious board
- selection as an expert representative for one's colleagues at a think tank

Achieving one of these milestones is a life-changing dynamic and, in the majority of instances, is due to an ever-evolving process of networking with colleagues and receiving mentoring, precepting, and coaching from advisers, role models, teachers, and others. Individuals interested in gaining these honors need to connect with others, and this needs to occur several times each year via e-mail, phone, or in person.

Shea and Gianotti (2009) describe mentoring as a progressive, mutually rewarding relationship where the mentor helps the mentee acquire knowledge and skills regarding his or her career, and the mentor also obtains benefits from the mentee. This may be a good universal definition because no mention is made of who matched the two people, no time limit is stated, and it allows both mentor and mentee to assist each other without the evaluation component hindering self-expression and growth for the sake of personal growth. However, the definition should be expanded to include more of a network of experts and probably have some formative evaluation built in. Furthermore, Shea and Gianotti define a mentor as someone having a positive effect on another and who goes above and beyond the job expectations. They define the mentee as an individual who uses the mentor's guidance and takes advantage of the mentor's advice.

The less skilled person in the classic mentoring relationship is called a *mentee, protégé,* or *novice,* whereas the more experienced is always alled a *mentor*. In order for the mentoring to be successful, Zachary (2009) suggests that the mentor have faith that the effective mentee will succeed. Motivation and empowerment generate mentoring, where both the mentor and mentee share their skills. In order to have an effective mentoring relationship, the mentor must try to remove obstacles, give emotional support, and allow for recognition of achievement in the work setting. In this way, mentees are encouraged to work harder to achieve their goals and ultimately achieve higher self-esteem as well. Being motivated to do a good job empowers the nurse, and this power makes the mentee feel motivated and confident to accomplish goals and gain increased self-esteem. The classic mentoring process is generally thought of as a relationship of two people: one (the mentee) who is a young and inexperienced person with great promise and the other who is a successful leader (the mentor) in the mentee's professional area. The mentor advises, teaches, coaches, role models, and connects the mentee to significant networks. Additionally, the mentee often needs to be able to offer a new skill set, resources, or some connection to the relationship that will benefit the mentor.

ADDITIONAL SUPPORT ROLES INVOLVED IN MENTORING

There are multiple perceptions about the roles of a mentor and mentee, what they involve, and what the differences are between a preceptor/preceptee or coach/apprentice relationship and the aforementioned mentor/mentee. Mentoring, in fact, is quite different from coaching (training for a project, executive role, or being on a task force), role modeling (this occurs often without any relationship between two individuals and often the role model does not know someone thinks he or she is a role model), or consulting (generally an outsider who is paid to do a part of a project or coordinate a project).

The roles are used interchangeably. Certainly everyone knows that the essence of what is being referred to here is that one person advises and coaches another person. So why is it necessary to operationally define mentoring, precepting, coaching, shadowing, or role modeling? Perhaps by defining these roles, people can have a better understanding of what type of guided experience would best fit the circumstances of the situation. Also, it seems prudent to provide a discussion of what is actually known about all of these terms, allowing research then to further validate each concept, so more appropriate guided experiences can be arranged for those who may or may not be able to experience a classic mentoring relationship.

Precepting

Preceptorships are generally used in health care, either with new nurse employees or nurses who are transitioning to new units, to orient them to their positions and responsibilities (Carlson, Pihammar, & Wann-Hansson, 2010). Precepting is also the format used when a student is assigned to a teacher, nurse, or some other experienced professional to teach this person as well as evaluate aspects of his or her role. The preceptor and preceptee are generally assigned by the patient care manager of the unit or by a faculty member. In nursing, a senior student generally has a preceptor in the clinical area that he or she is assigned to work with for approximately 160 hours in the student's final semester. This model is also used for graduate nursing students who are assigned to a preceptor for a clinical rotation. The student follows the preceptor's schedule and works in a one-to-one relationship for a specific amount of time. The student has a faculty member who makes regular visits or some type of contact with the preceptor, to assess how the preceptee is doing and discuss the student's performance on a routine basis. The preceptor is responsible to evaluate the student on a pass/fail checklist and reviews this with the student and faculty at the end of the required number of hours in the preceptorship. Experiential learning has been the mainstay of professional internships in most disciplines and used to teach not only the professional practice skills but also how to communicate and affect change in one's practice (Kolb, 1984).

Coaching

One function of a mentor is to coach the mentee by keeping the mentee aware of the politics in the organization, being supportive of the person's ideas, and acting as a sounding board when the mentee needs to discuss how to overcome weaknesses. Gilley and Boughton (2004) say the key to maximizing organizational performance is to have work environments that allow for increased self-esteem of all employees and provide not only for accomplishing organizational goals but also personal growth and development. Coaching can be defined as comprising four roles: training, career coaching, confronting, and mentoring. The most important of these to the organization is the confronter role, which includes learning to be assertive, managing conflict, and collaborating to solve organizational problems. The faculty person is the coach in the student-preceptor-coach triangle and is responsible for obtaining the correct experiences and opportunities, so that the student can accomplish individual and program goals.

Boreen and Niday (2003) also suggest the notion of self-mentoring or coaching oneself toward growth that others may refer to as auto-mentoring. Strategies used are reflection techniques, motivational self-talk, questioning, listening, critical thinking, and risk taking. Keeping weekly logs of positive and negative occurrences, discussing different ways to handle negative incidents, and implementing these new strategies facilitate the self-mentoring process. It is also important to have a network of peers to bounce ideas off of and share solutions for negative experiences. Self-reflection assists individuals to increase self-awareness and reprioritize their needs in order to maximize growth. Mentoring has proven to be one of the most effective ways to keep teachers in the field, and this is thought to be true in the nursing profession as well.

Reciprocity

In shadowing or role modeling, there is generally an aspect of closeness between the role model and the individual, although it is not uncommon for the role model to be totally unaware that someone is actually seeing him or her as a role model. Each of these role-modeling relationships has a place in assisting individuals to grow both professionally and personally. Role modeling is defined as extremely important in order to succeed with human adaptation (Kolb, 1984, 2000). It facilitates learning by offering behaviors that the less experienced person can imitate. Many times this imitation is specific to one type of behavior that a role model exemplifies. Other times, people imitate role models for a general look or response that they perceive would be helpful to adapt in their own professional and personal growth. Experiential learning has been the mainstay of professional internships in most disciplines and used to teach not only professional practice skills but also how to communicate and effect change in one's practice (Kolb, 1984).

COMPONENTS OF THE MENTORING PROCESS

Zachary (2009) summarizes the components of the mentor–mentee relationship as including reciprocity, collaboration, partnership, mutually defined goals, learning, and development for both the mentor and the mentee. Although the major focus of this section will be on the mentoring process, there will be some discussion on how precepting and coaching relate to the components.

Reciprocity

Most all agree that there is some degree of benefit for the mentor as well as the mentee. Many often ask "What's in it for me to meet and assist someone with their career?" With the more expanded view of mentoring, it does seem that more people are agreeing to mentor. They see that they will benefit from connecting with their mentee's mentoring network via the mentee as well as directly gain from the mentee. Here, reciprocity is the "give and take" that occurs between the mentor and mentee.

Collaboration and Partnership

Higgins and Kram (2001) found that almost all professionals have a developmental network of people who mentor them. The networks include junior, peer, and senior professionals as well as family and friends. Bunker, Hall, and Kram (2010) emphasize the importance of partnering with other health care agencies and interdisciplinary collaboration. If a specific skill is identified as something the mentee needs to acquire, this is when the mentor or, more aptly, the mentee, can reach out to connect with someone to teach the mentee, such as a coach who can meet over a specific period of time to train the mentee or a preceptor, who the mentee works alongside of to master a specific skill.

Mutually Defined Goals

Both the mentor and mentee should identify separately their goals and motives for the mentor–mentee relationship in operational terms and with target dates, and commit to a mutually beneficial relationship (Metros & Yang, 2005). It is also important to decide whether or not the mentor plans to delegate part of her or his job to the mentee, and if the mentee plans to progress within the organization after the mentorship or plans to move to another organization. Plans for obtaining skills and knowledge for the mentee that the mentor cannot give also should be created with other mentors, preceptors, or coaches. Hogue and Pringle (2005) developed the following principles to assist in developing goals for a mentor–mentee relationship: work for mutual benefits, be confidential with all that occurs in the mentorship, practice honesty consistently, take time to hear both sides and learn from this, develop a genuine and respectful relationship, role play leading, and practice flexibility.

Learning

This component speaks to what the mentoring process is supposedly going to increase for the mentee—all of the knowledge, experience, skills, and exposure to the "right" network of professionals who are working in similar areas as the mentee. This is what the mentor and mentee will be creating goals to obtain.

Development of Both the Mentor and Mentee

This component includes the various developmental milestones that the mentor and mentee accomplish with their relationship and their own goal attainment through this relationship, along with the larger mentoring network that has been created.

Relationship

The relationship between the mentor and mentee will be what they create. It can span the continuum of class dyads to a multiple mentoring relationship, where a person has multiple mentors who are their peers, superiors, or even their underlings. This relationship can be formal or informal, and can involve preceptor and coach. Clearly, there is a spectrum of interactions that will dictate the type of relationship needed for success, depending on the situation (see Figure 1.1). The horizontal continuum shows formal relatedness (a structured agreement that meets the mentor and mentee's goals) to the extreme left of the continuum and an informal relatedness on the extreme right side of the continuum. Situational responses are isolated incidents of specific advising by an experienced or knowledgeable individual to meet another individual's needs. The formal aspect of this relatedness framework includes a formative and summative evaluation of the mentee, a proficiently completed job skill checklist for the preceptee, and an evaluation of growth by the coachee. The informal aspect of the framework includes the genuine caring that evolves between the mentor and mentee, a possible collegial bond between the preceptor and preceptee, and a potential friendliness that could develop between the coach and coachee.

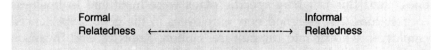

| Formal | Informal |
| Relatedness ←----------------------------------→ | Relatedness |

FIGURE 1.1   Continuum of Relatedness by the Mentor, Preceptor, and Coach

Kram (1986), a foremost classic mentoring expert, identifies three primary components of mentoring that are most frequently part of a mentorship. The psychosocial aspect includes assisting a person to acclimate to an organization's culture, suggesting hints for balancing work and personal life, whereas career focuses involve networking, providing strategies for accomplishing goals for career advancement, and new professional endeavors. Some mentoring relationships consist of assisting the mentee with personal development issues such as balancing family and career, moving to the right neighborhood, socializing with the politically correct crowd, dressing for the part, and vacationing at the correct places. These mentoring dyads tend to be long-term relationships that last for an extended period of time, or even forever. The mentor and mentee become friends and share a great amount of time together. Other mentorships leave the personal development area to the mentee to gain from others. The idea of developing trust between the mentor and mentee that increases with time is a significant part of the relationship, since it allows for support and sharing of experiences. The mentor's job includes career functions, such as sponsorship, coaching, protection, and exposure, while the psychosocial role involves role modeling, counseling, acceptance, confirmation, and friendship. Kram (1983) points out that not all of these functions may be appropriate in some organizations or with some individuals, but clarifies that a mentorship should include focusing on psychosocial issues as well as advising on steps for career advancement. It is not uncommon for a mentor and mentee to identify specific outcomes they expect to gain from the relationship. In some settings, contracts are developed that set out the expectations of each party.

RATIONALES FOR THE EMERGENCE OF CONTEMPORARY MENTORING

Human resource departments have been singing the praises of mentoring since the 1950s. When management clarified how important it was for employees to be tied to the organization and be loyal for the good of the organization, more and more employees were tagged as fitting into the culture or not. Administration was interested in cloning the "good ones," and this is where specific plans were instituted in business corporations that assigned new employees to the good, experienced employees who fit into the culture. Holton, Knowles, and Swanson (2011), master adult educators, have written about how adults learn and can relearn at any age. Business models, of course, are used in coaching new employees to become effective executives. Mentees can gain increased knowledge from their assigned mentors. Adult learners generally want to learn for learning's sake but there are a few who need assistance transitioning to facilitating their own learning versus being spoon fed and trained to please the teacher. There is a continuous movement of a more self-directed emphasis for learners to assume responsibility for their own growth and learning (Taylor, Marienau, & Fiddler, 2000). This includes the idea of setting up shadowing experiences with experts and having internships in which learners can practice their skills. Lifelong learning also triggered a self-development context in which individuals were guided to become more performance centered versus content focused. This paradigm change influenced educators to set up learning experiences in which the student had exposure to and practice time in the work he or she wanted to do after graduation. Given that the educator could not be in two places at the same time, students were assigned to work with individuals who worked in the specific area in which they needed experience. As such, the precepting model used in nursing, pharmacy, medicine, and other professional training programs was instituted.

Stoddard and Tamasy (2009) suggest that classic mentoring is a long-term involvement between two individuals. They emphasize that the mentor must be able to see the mentee as multidimensional and always changing. Additionally, they feel that a "true" mentorship goes way beyond teaching someone skills, and must take on a holistic relationship; thus, dealing with all aspects of the mentee's needs. The mentor is believed to facilitate the mentee in developing skills and acquiring networks and organizational savvy that is crucial for survival as well as success in any profession. Others argue (Sinetar, 1998; Weil, 2001) that mentoring relationships evolve over time, are spontaneous and not assigned, and tend to be critical for leadership succession in any profession. So it seems there is disagreement as to whether mentoring must evolve over time or exist for a specified time period, whether a spontaneous connection can prompt a mentoring dyad, and whether mentors should formally evaluate a mentee. The emergence of new mentoring models, such as multiple mentors, the junior partner reciprocally mentoring the senior individual, and peer mentoring networks are all products of the classic mentor–mentee dyad.

TYPES OF MENTORING

Multiple Mentoring

Mentoring is a complex relationship between two people, and the process is even more complex when the mentee, mentor, or both are involved in more than one mentoring relationship. This simultaneous mentoring involvement, called *multiple mentoring*, has become more common as the Internet and communication technology have allowed more global and quick connections. For example, in a multiple mentoring model, the mentee can seek out advice from more than one mentor as well as use the most qualified mentor for each need. *Reverse mentoring* is when a senior person receives mentoring from a junior person or the mentor is mentored by the mentee. An example of this reverse mentoring follows:

Susan, a doctoral student, has begun a mentorship with Dr. Theng, who studies the concept of hardiness in chronic illness. Susan has been receiving hints and suggestions, such as which conferences to submit abstracts for presentation, whether to submit for a paper or poster presentation, ideas on PowerPoint and poster development, and strategies for being chosen to keynote a conference or be a part of a symposium or panel, and has even been connected to Dr. Theng's collegial network as she prepares for a presentation she is doing with Dr. Theng at a national conference. Susan suggests to Dr. Theng that they incorporate web enhancement technology in the presentation. Dr. Theng is not familiar with Starboard Technology, and so Susan shares her expertise with her mentor. Dr. Theng is elated with the results and has Susan assist her in making these applications to all of her class presentations. Susan also has 10 years of experience working as a diabetic teaching nurse and 5 years of experience working as a family nurse practitioner. She has access to all patient data files in the clinic, which includes over 6,000 chronically ill people. She is still a per diem practitioner at this clinic and has received Institutional Review Board consent to study hardiness with diabetics. Using this database, she is going to be working as the primary researcher with Dr. Theng as a co-investigator.

This example portrays the give-and-take relationship that often occurs in nursing, in which most individuals have clinical expertise and a network in an area prior to returning for a higher degree. They come to the mentoring relationship to gain knowledge and experience in administration, education, or research.

Peer and Co-Mentoring

Co-mentoring or peer mentoring is dependent on mutual trust and is similar to traditional mentoring in that way; however, it differs greatly with regard to equality. Since there is no hierarchical relationship, the colleagues must be extremely trustworthy of each other so that neither of them derives more or less from the connection. Another benefit of peer mentoring is the teaching and leadership that peer mentors can provide to the mentee and the organization (Hunt & Ellison, 2010). An example of this is the Peer Mentoring Program initiated at a western Ontario university in their nursing laboratory, which also assisted in decreasing costs (Dennison, 2010).

Rymer (2002) and Sinetar (1998) reinforce the significance of each individual having equal roles in peer mentoring. It is a myth that only elders or organizational superiors can be mentors. In fact, Sinetar (1998) goes as far as to say that any virtuous energy, including a friend, a child, or an idea, can mentor or inspire us. All of these models assist with acclimating mentees to their jobs and advancing their career paths, as well as helping their mentor's career.

With the multiple mentoring and reverse mentoring models, horizontal and vertical mentoring can occur simultaneously, depending on a variety of beneficial and mitigating factors. For example, there are mixed results on what type of mentoring functions are best to ensure gender and cultural diversity between mentor and mentee (Clutterbuck & Ragins, 2002).

Sue's (1981) Minority Identity Model, which explains how minorities progress through five psychosocial stages of cultural identity development as they work with a mentor, exemplifies a successful model in this regard. The five psychosocial stages follow:

- *Conformity.* The individual tends to be self-deprecating and relates to his or her own culture.
- *Dissonance.* The person is developing some conflict with the culture.
- *Resistance and immersion.* The individual is more self-deprecating and is rejecting the dominant society.
- *Introspection.* There is much self-evaluation and reflection for the dominant society and how the person is interacting.
- *Synergism and awareness.* The individual can accept his or her own cultural identity but also develops a selective appreciation of the culture in which he or she is currently immersed.

What are the implications of these stages to mentoring? It depends where the individual is in identity development; thus, mentees have different needs depending on what stage they are experiencing. This can be compounded if the mentor and the mentee are of the same culture but are in different stages of the identity model. This is where the mentor will need to role model well regarding the importance for a mentee to find or develop his or her own style and not conform to the style of another. It is important to be aware of the issue of cultural diversity, and to try to use the developmental framework already noted or a similar model to educate both the mentor and mentee, so appropriate networking and advisement can be ensured. If a structured mentoring program is in effect, it is helpful to have opportunities to involve culturally diverse individuals so as to maximize networking with others.

Schwiebert (2000) indicates there are not enough mentors for all who seek one, especially for culturally diverse individuals. She points out that there are many mentors who practice alterity, which is the perpetuation of a monocultural concept of mentoring. It is when one person truly believes that anyone outside his or her own culture is strange or inferior, and so feels that he or she should set the standards for all people. This would obviously thwart mentoring success for many individuals, especially those from minority groups. It is not known if pairing mentor and mentee with a similar cultural background has the optimum outcome. Depending on the awareness of the mentor, there could be serious misunderstandings transferred to the mentee, which can often result from insensitivity and ignorance (Schwiebert, 2000). The question remains: If no culturally similar mentor can be found for a mentee, is it better to have no mentor or one from a different culture? Further research on transcultural mentoring is necessary in all disciplines.

Peers, peer pals, co-mentors, and *buddies* are terms given for collaborative mentoring relationships between peers. These groups of colleagues are generally noncompetitive and are willing to network with each other to accomplish mutually agreed-on goals.

Daloz (1999) describes an individual's education as a transformational journey affected by mentor guides who model, offer a map, conceptualize, and provide a mirror. He correlates mentoring with teaching in that few teachers ever have the privilege of following a student through the entire journey but instead tend to accompany students along some parts of their journeys.

Miller (2002) describes various examples of co-mentoring, interning, role modeling, and coaching. He presents two case studies depicting mentoring with Deloitte and Touche and Merrill Lynch's Scholarship Builder Program. He believes that mentoring in the business world is seen as important as work experience in an employee's career development and that it will continue to be appreciated even if a mentor and mentee are not in close geographic proximity. Telementoring and e-mail mentoring are becoming common tools used especially among peer networks and multiple mentoring relationships in business.

CHARACTERISTICS OF THE CLASSIC MENTORING RELATIONSHIP

Wilson and Elman (1990) believe that mentoring is the most successful way to pass along the "norms, values, assumptions, and myths that are central to an organization's survival" (p. 93). As a dynamic process, mentoring is continuing to evolve, so it becomes easier for important legacies and an organization's values to be passed on to the next generation. So, too, with a nursing mentor-mentee relationship, the values or beliefs of the profession can be preserved.

The classic, formal mentoring dyad generally lasts for about 5 to 10 years (Kram, 1986; Levinson et al., 1978). Be that as it may, our current long-term mentoring is assigned and generally lasts for a period sufficient for the mentee or preceptee to learn the skills appropriate for a position. Informal mentoring, of course, is spontaneous and nonassigned. Interestingly, Kram (1986) found that with formal mentoring there is more superficiality between mentor and mentee than in an informal relationship.

Wickman and Sjodin (1996) describe many interesting accounts of their mentoring relationship, which lasted about 5 years, in which Wickman was generally the mentor and Sjodin was generally the mentee. Their book, *Mentoring: The Most Obvious Yet Overlooked Key to Achieving More in Life Than You Ever Dreamed Possible,* is helpful in explaining exactly how to go about getting a mentor or advising someone else interested in obtaining a mentor as well as strategies for maximizing the benefits of a mentoring relationship.

STAGES OF THE MENTORING PROCESS

Kram's (1983) longitudinal study of mentor–mentee pairs in business found certain similarities between the pairs that helped identify the phases of the mentoring process. She found most relationships averaged 5 years in length and consisted of four stages. Others have validated this research in both business (Ensher & Murphy, 2011) and education settings (Pask & Joy, 2007). Stages include:

1. *Initiation stage.* The senior person is admired, and the junior person is considered coachable, and a general getting-to-know-each-other time begins.

2. *Cultivation stage.* The mentee is at the peak of development, sets goals, and gains self-esteem, and generally works on both professional and personal goal achievement.
3. *Separation stage.* The junior person starts to express independence. It is a time of anxiety when the junior person separates from the senior person. The intensity in the relationship begins to decrease considerably.
4. *Redefinition stage.* There is a collegial relationship that allows for more equality between the mentee and the mentor. The mentee may feel abandoned, depending on where he or she is developmentally. It is the time that most feel the relationship is no longer needed or desired, or it becomes a more peer-like relationship (Kram, 1983).

These stages of mentoring portray a cyclical process or a continuum that is based on the individual's developmental stages as he or she matures in the relationship. Depending on where one is in one's life and career, one will generally be either mentoring someone, be mentored, or be in a network that co-mentors one another. When one reviews stages of the mentoring process, it is most common to think of Kram's (1983) universal stages.

However, it might be important to also factor into this framework the idea that mentors may mentor differently depending on where they are in developing their mentoring skills. Most mentors are made, not born, and that is why it is interesting to review Bennis's framework. Mentoring is part of being a leader and, similar to developing one's leadership ability, one will need to build mentoring skills.

Bennis (2004) likens the stages that leaders go through to the seven ages of man as described by Shakespeare in *As You Like It*. Bennis describes the mentoring a leader experiences as the leader evolves:

- *Stage 1, Infant Executive.* It is crucial that during this stage, the infant executive has a mentor. Bennis says that a mentor has attributes of both male and female gender, which points to the potential richness of the relationship and suggests that a mentor relationship is deeper than just a teacher and student. In reality "mentors do not materialize on their own" (p. 48); rather, the best mentors are "usually recruited." A characteristic of a true leader is having the ability to "identify, woo, and win the mentors who will change his/her life" (p. 48). This is comparable to the ability of an experienced head-hunter who gets a client placed.
- *Stage 2, Schoolboy With Shining Face.* The new leader should "make a low-key entry" while he or she learns the culture and benefits

from the wisdom of those already there. It is imperative for a mentee to "establish [being] open to the contributions of others."

- *Stage 3, Lover, With a Woeful Ballad.* This is the time when one needs to separate from colleagues as friends since they are no longer one's peers. It becomes crucial to delegate.
- *Stage 4, Beautiful Soldier.* The mentor may become too comfortable with his or her role. The mentor should be sure to nurture his or her shining stars, but not take from them without due recognition.
- *Stage 5, General, Full of Wise Saws.* It is crucial to hear both the good and the bad and to act accordingly.
- *Stage 6, Statesman With Spectacles on Nose.* It is here one should do more mentoring since this is when a leader's power base wanes.
- *Stage 7, Sage, Second Childishness.* This is where having mentored throughout one's career will pay off. It is the professional equivalent of having grandchildren and leaving a legacy for future generations.

Bennis says each stage of leadership a person experiences in life brings new crises and challenges, and that having experienced these stages, one then knows what to expect, and this knowledge allows one to help not only oneself but also others to get through life's challenges. Similarly, one can envision how a nurse would follow various mentors' steps during his or her nursing career.

ADVANTAGES AND DISADVANTAGES OF MENTORING

Many (Bell, 1998; Bennetts, 2000; Sinetar, 1998) identify benefits for the mentee, mentor, and organization, including

- quicker learning curves for mentee and mentor
- increased communication of corporate values
- reduced turnover at a time when new recruits may be difficult to locate
- increased loyalty
- improved one-on-one communication and team spirit within work groups
- increased employee productivity
- added time for oneself to work on one's own goals
- added information from mentees regarding what is going on outside your department
- creation of allies in the mentees for the future

These advantages are helpful to the mentor, mentee, organization, and the profession. Peluchete and Jeanquart (2000) describe the impact mentors have by connecting students and novices to the correct person for career success. Another advantage for mentors is that by mentoring, they develop increased credibility in the organization (Gilley & Boughton, 1996). One can gain credibility by delegating work appropriately, providing specific and timely performance feedback, helping employees identify work objectives for improvement, and demonstrating acceptable professional behavior.

Sinetar (1998) warns there are disadvantages of mentoring if "unhealthy mentors" attempt to manipulate mentees. Certainly it is possible for mentors to treat mentees without dignity and respect. Although the mentors may appear ultra-aggressive and confident, usually these mentors are intimidated and have very low self-esteem. Therefore, these types of individuals should be quickly identified as unsuitable mentors who are actually in need of a mentor—or at least guidance—for themselves. People who are this insecure at a later stage of their careers may not be candidates for participating in a mentoring partnership since they cannot share and will do too much harm to their mentors or their mentees and themselves. There are also individuals who have been mentored and helped along the way who do not have any realization of it at all, or at least cannot admit that they have been mentored and have not climbed the ladder solely on their own. These individuals should not be tapped as mentors either.

There are other disadvantages as well, such as personality incompatibility, power-mongering mentors, and situations in which mentors are resentful of their mentees and make trouble for them that can sabotage their careers. Simon and Eby (2003) present findings that provide a description of negative mentoring experiences that they have collected. These relationships can vary in severity and frequency and may be characterized by minor obstructionism (e.g., not returning phone calls), hostility (e.g., talking negatively about someone behind his or her back), or serious overt aggression (e.g., physical attack). Possessiveness, jealousy, credit taking, deceit, and abuse, both psychological and physical, can occur in mentoring relationships.

CONCLUSION

As one realizes the significance that mentoring can have on some individuals, it becomes more readily understood that perhaps there is something to what people say when they describe their mentorship: "I still think about things we used to discuss or I try to think how my mentor would manage a challenge facing me, and it has been 17 years." "I still, after 21 years, use things that I learned from my mentoring experience, and I feel good when something triggers me to remember these 'lessons.'" Both Siegel (2010) and Siegel (2007) study the neurology of interpersonal relationships and write about how we become the people we are through our interpersonal connections and reflective thoughts. They elaborate that the mind emerges from the brain and its structures and that functions of the brain are directly shaped by interpersonal relationships. Due to the connection between the brain structure and its function, research has provided new insights into how experience and mindful awareness increases physiological benefits such as in our immune and cardiac functions, and also develops the prefrontal cortex. By further developing the prefrontal cortex, we are able to increase neural circuits or expand our neuroplasticity, which allows us to increase our ability to think and learn. So there is more evidence that having a mentor or mentors, a preceptor, or coach has a significant impact on humans, and the wisdom and shared learning one can gain from these individuals has a positive influence on our ability to engage in interpersonal relationships throughout life.

The idea of providing mentorships prevails in practice disciplines such as education, business, and nursing. There are opportunities from using best practices in mentoring to:

- develop new models of support for people to succeed
- maximize creative recruitment and retention strategies for the organization
- strengthen the profession by producing increased knowledge and theory

It is becoming more and more evident that teachers and students, supervisors and subordinates, managers and staff, and peers with colleagues are being successful in advancing individual, organizational, and professional goals with mentoring. Also, there is no one way of mentoring. It is important that the various terms used to describe a mentoring process be defined operationally so that individuals have clarity when reading results of research, setting up mentoring programs, and describing their own mentoring experience.

This mentoring experience comprises a skill/content and a psychosocial support component. Most significant, people need to understand the type of relationship that has occurred and how this relationship served the mentor, mentee, organization, and profession. It is realistic for most people to have more than one mentoring experience in their lives and also work with multiple preceptors, coaches, and role models. If someone is fortunate enough to have a long-term mentoring relationship, then this is a classic mentor–mentee relationship. It is in this case that the two individuals willingly spend time together as they share experiences and learn from each other.

Sheehy (2006) calls this partnership that develops over time the *mentor connection* and refers to it as a successful linking. Findings that support positive outcomes from the preceptor, coach, and role model relationships also support success. There is general consensus that individuals who have or have had good mentoring relationships tend to be well balanced with personal and work issues as well as successful in their professional careers. More research identifying best practices in mentoring will serve to accentuate the need for a mentoring culture within and between disciplines.

REFERENCES

Andrews, M., & Wallis, M. (1999). Mentorship in nursing: A literature review. *Journal of Advanced Nursing, 29*, 201–207.

Bell, C. (1998). *Managers as mentors: Building partnerships for learning* (2nd ed.). San Francisco, CA: Berrett-Koehler.

Bennetts, C. (2000). The traditional mentor relationship and the well being of creative individuals in school and work. *International Journal of Health Promotion and Education, 38*, 22–27.

Bennis, W. (2004). The seven ages of the leader. *Harvard Business Review, 82*, 46–53.

Boreen, J., & Niday, D. (2003). *Mentoring across boundaries: Helping beginning teachers succeed in challenging situations.* Portland, ME: Stenhouse.

Bunker, K. A., Hall, D. T., & Kram, K. E. (2010). *Extraordinary leadership.* San Francisco, CA: Jossey-Bass.

Carlson, E., Pilhammar, E., & Wann-Hansson, C. (2010). Time to precept: Supportive and limiting conditions for precepting nurses. *Journal of Advanced Nursing, 66*(2), 432–441.

Clutterbuck, D., & Ragins, B. R. (2002). *Mentoring and diversity: An international perspective.* Oxford, England: Butterworth-Heinemann.

Cottrell, D. (2006). *Monday morning mentoring: Ten lessons to guide you up the ladder.* New York, NY: HarperCollins Publishers.

Daloz, L. (1999). *Mentor: Guiding the journey of adult learners* (2nd ed.). San Francisco, CA: Jossey-Bass.

Dennison, S. (2010). Peer mentoring: Untapped potential. *Journal of Nursing Education, 49*(6), 340–342.

Dungy, T. (2010). *The mentor leader: Secrets to building people and teams that win consistently.* Winter Park, FL: Legacy, LLC.

Ensher, E. A., & Murphy, S. E. (2011). *Power mentoring: How successful mentors and protégés get the most out of their relationships.* San Francisco, CA: Jossey-Bass.

Fenelon, F. (1994). *Les aventures de Telemaque [The adventures of Telemachus]* (P. Riley, Trans.). Cambridge: Cambridge University Press. (Original work published 1699.)

Gay, B. (1994). What is mentoring? *Education and Training, 36,* 4–7.

Gilley, J., & Boughton, N. (1996). *Stop managing, start coaching!: How performance coaching can enhance commitment and improve productivity.* New York, NY: McGraw-Hill.

Higgins, M. C., & Kram, K. E. (2001). Reconceptualizing mentoring at work: A developmental network perspective. *Academy of Management Review, 2* (26), 264–288.

Hogue, W., & Pringle, E. (2005). What's next after you say hello: First steps in mentoring. *EDUCAUSE Quarterly, 26*(2), 50–52.

Holton, E. F., Knowles, M., & Swanson, R. A. (2011). *The adult learner: The definitive classic in adult education and human resource development* (7th ed.). San Francisco, CA: Jossey-Bass.

Homer. (1946). *The odyssey* (E. V. Rieu, Trans.). Harmondsworth, England: Penguin.

Hunt, C. W., & Ellison, K. J. (2010). Enhancing faculty resources through peer mentoring. *Nurse Educator, 35*(5), 192–196.

Jonson, K.F. (2008). *Being an effective mentor: How to help beginning teachers succeed* (2nd ed.). Thousand Oaks, CA: Corwin Press.

Kolb, D. (1984). *Experiential learning.* Englewood Cliffs, NJ: Prentice Hall.

Kolb, D. (2000). *Facilitator's guide to learning.* Boston, MA: Hay/McBer Training Resources Group.

Kram, K. (1983). Phases of the mentor relationship. *Academy of Management Journal, 26,* 608–625.

Kram, K. (1986). Mentoring in the workplace. In D. Hall (Ed.), *Career development in organizations.* San Francisco, CA: Jossey-Bass.

Levinson, D., Darrow, E., Klein, M., Levinson, M., & McKee, B. (1978). *The seasons of a man's life.* New York, NY: Knopf.

Luna, G., & Cullen, D. (2000). *Empowering the faculty: Mentoring redirected and renewed.* Washington, DC: George Washington University Press.

Maxwell, J.C. (2008). *Mentoring 101: What every leader needs to know.* Nashville, TN: Thomas Nelson.

McWeeny, M. (2002). The changing mosaic of mentoring. *Creative Nursing Journal, 3,* 3–4.

Metros, S. E., & Yang, C. (2005). The importance of mentors. In C. Golden (Ed.), *Cultivating careers* (Chapter 5, Educause). Retrieved from http://www.educause.edu/Resources/CultivatingCareersProfessional/Chapter5TheImportanceofMentors/10631

Miller, A. (2002). *Mentoring students and young people.* Sterling, VA: Stylus Publishing.

Murray, M. (2001). *Beyond the myths and magic of mentoring: How to facilitate an effective mentoring process* (2nd ed.). San Francisco, CA: Jossey-Bass.

National Post. (2007, July 4). *The second fastest growing profession.* Retrieved from http://www.canada.com/nationalpost/financialpost/story.html?id=eac6cc01-509b-4141-bd61-a0614888ef14

Pask, R., & Joy, B. (2007). *Mentoring–coaching: A guide for educational professionals.* New York, NY: McGraw-Hill.

Peluchete, J., & Jeanquart, S. (2000). Professionals' use of different mentor sources at various career stages: Implications for career success. *Journal of Social Psychology, 140,* 549–564.

Ragins, K. A., & Kram, K. E. (Eds.) (2007). *The handbook of mentoring at work* (2nd ed.). Thousand Oaks, CA: Sage Publications Inc.

Roberts, A. (2000). Mentoring revisited: A phenomenological reading of the literature. *Mentoring and Tutoring, 8,* 145–170.

Rymer, J. (2002). "Only connect": Transforming ourselves and our discipline through co-mentoring. *Journal of Business Communication, 39,* 342–364.

Schweibert, V. (2000). *Mentoring: Creating connected, empowered relationships.* Alexandria, VA: American Counseling Association.

Shea, G. F., & Gianotti, S. C. (2009). *Mentoring: Make it a mutually rewarding experience.* Menlo Park, CA: Crisp Learning.

Sheehy, G. (2006). *Passages: Predictable crises of adult life.* New York, NY: Random House, Inc.

Siegel, D. (2007). *The mindful brain: Reflection and attunement in the cultivation of well-being.* New York, NY: W.W. Norton & Company, Inc.

Siegel, R. D. (2010). *The mindfulness solution: Everyday practices for everyday problems.* New York, NY: Guilford Press.

Simon, S., & Eby, L. (2003). A typology of negative mentoring experiences: A multidimensional scaling study. *Human Relations, 56,* 1083–1106.

Sinetar, M. (1998). *The mentor's spirit: Life lessons on leadership and the art of encouragement.* New York, NY: St. Martin's Press.

Sommers-Flanagan, R., & Sommers-Flanagan, J. (2007). *Becoming an ethical helping professional: Cultural and philosophical foundation.* Hoboken, NJ: John Wiley & Sons, Inc.

Stoddard, D. A., & Tamasy, R. J. (2009). *The heart of mentoring: Ten proven principles.* Colorado Springs, CO: NavPress.

Strike, K. T., & Nickerson, J. (2011). *Mentoring the educational leader: A practical framework for success.* Blue Ridge Summit, PA: Rowman & Littlefield Education.

Sue, D. (1981). *Counseling the culturally different.* New York, NY: Wiley.

Taylor, K., Marineau, C. & Fiddler, M. (2000). *Developing adult learners: Strategies for teachers.* San Francisco, CA: Jossey-Bass.

University of New Mexico Mentoring Institute and International Mentoring Association. (2011). *Learning across disciplines.* Retrieved January 27, 2012, from http://mentor.unm.edu/conference/index.html.

Weil, V. (2001). Mentoring: Some ethical considerations. *Science and Engineering Ethics, 7,* 471–482.

Wickman, F., & Sjodin, T. (1996). *Mentoring: The most obvious yet overlooked key to achieving more in life than you ever dreamed possible.* New York, NY: McGraw-Hill.

Wilson, J., & Elman, N. (1990). Organizational benefits of mentoring. *Academy of Management Executive, 4,* 88–94.

Zachary, L. (2005). *Creating a mentoring culture: The organization's guide.* San Francisco, CA: Jossey-Bass.

Zachary, L. (2009). *The mentee's guide: Making mentoring work for you.* San Francisco, CA: Jossey-Bass.

2

A Mentoring Culture for Nurses

DEFINITION OF MENTORING IN NURSING

Reviewing descriptions of mentoring, precepting, and coaching from disciplines outside nursing in Chapter 1 will have hopefully increased our knowledge regarding how mentoring has developed in the nursing profession to support the following definition: Mentoring in nursing encompasses a guided, reciprocal, formal or informal, evaluated experience, assigned or prearranged over a mutually agreed-on period of time that empowers the mentor and mentee to develop personally and professionally within the auspices of a caring, collaborative, and respectful environment. Having an understanding of the differences between mentoring, precepting, and coaching will assist in validating how mentoring has expanded and evolved from a classic dyad to a dynamic network.

For example, if a new junior faculty member, Robert, establishes a classic mentorship with the senior faculty member in his area, Ron, but needs time orienting to the nearby hospital in Labor & Delivery so he can do clinical teaching and practice in the unit, then a preceptorship for Robert will be set up with an experienced staff nurse on the Labor & Delivery Unit. This preceptor will orient and precept Robert so he will be able to be a staff nurse and also a clinical faculty member on the Labor & Delivery Unit but then his relationship with the preceptor will most likely stop. Robert will continue to be mentored by Ron for a few years or perhaps longer. During this mentorship, it is most likely Ron who will connect Robert with other experienced individuals or coaches who will assist Robert in familiarizing himself with many different skills and experiences. Robert will eventually be a mentee in a multiple mentoring model and perhaps mentor others as well in some areas.

Nursing needs to develop a mentoring culture; that is, all nurses should experience being in a collaborative network that fosters partnering with others. Most nurses today receive precepting during their orientation to a clinical position or coaching for a special project or promotion they are preparing for, or perhaps they look up to someone as a role model who inspires them. But most do not have experience in a classic mentoring dyad or group. Some have also had coaching relationships with people who have taught them a skill or assisted them with college admissions or career planning. The majority of individuals in the nursing profession who have had mentoring are doctorally prepared nurses with their dissertation chair, along with some fortunate middle managers in service who may be mentored by their senior nurse administrators. With the new mentoring models such as peer and multiple mentoring, every nurse could benefit from being in a mentoring culture. Indeed, this culture should permeate the nursing workforce for broader impact, not only with individual nurses who desire mentoring but also within the organization and the profession. This becomes more pressing when considering the emerging workforce: ever more master's-prepared nurses in their 20s. In fact, the profession needs to adapt the "mentoring relationships lineage model," as conducted by Jack Welch and the team of General Electric (GE), where the GE mentoring culture is available to employees and especially those interested in executive careers (Ensher & Murphy, 2011). If everyone took mentoring seriously and felt it was their responsibility to bring up the junior employees just coming in, there would be more self-empowerment and increased self-confidence in future leaders. This chapter thus describes nursing's vision of the development of a mentoring culture.

The following definition of *mentoring* emerges from the literature on descriptions of mentoring: Mentoring in nursing encompasses a guided experience, formally or informally assigned, over a mutually agreed-on period, that empowers the mentor and mentee to develop personally and professionally within the auspices of a caring, collaborative, culturally competent, and respectful environment. Evidence-based mentoring practice in nursing can support each component of this definition.

A Guided Experience

Mentor is often used interchangeably with *preceptor, coach, assessor, teacher/supervisor,* and *adviser.* Stewart and Krueger (1996), however, distinguish separate processes here. A *preceptor* is assigned to work alongside and evaluate new employees, a *coach* gives skill-training tips on a regular basis, an *assessor* evaluates the employee's performance, the *teacher/supervisor* facilitates new opportunities to increase the person's knowledge and experiential base and acts as a resource, and the *adviser* suggests specific strategies to obtain a degree or advance one's career. In England, *mentor* is identified as being synonymous with *preceptor, supervisor,* and *assessor* (Andrews & Wallis, 1999). The classic term *mentoring* is thus loosely used in the nursing profession, and includes each of the roles mentioned that one experienced individual will assume with a less experienced individual, over a mutually determined period of time. Stewart and Krueger (1996) also studied related concepts of mentoring such as role modeling, sponsoring, precepting, peer strategizing, collaborating, and coaching. Table 2.1 compares and contrasts the definition of these terms during the 1990s through 2012.

There has been some change in the perception of mentoring and its related roles over the past decade in that co-mentoring and multiple mentoring have greatly increased. There is a great deal of research on the increase in mentoring in the purest sense in doctoral education. Precepting remains the most frequently cited aspect of "mentoring" for nurses today, and it involves assigned relationships with students or new orienting nurses and experienced nurses in a time-limited and evaluation-oriented experience.

Formal Versus Informal Assignments: Stages of the Mentoring Process

Mentoring is considered best when it occurs spontaneously (or is unassigned) between two people (Restifo & Yoder, 2004). There is more informal matching that occurs, and sometimes this mentoring does not continue over an extended period of time. Most nurses have assigned precepting experiences for their orientation to a new unit. Some may ask the preceptor to be their mentor when their orientation comes to a close. Still others network with peers and mentor each other during orientation or a specific course. Andrews and Wallis (1999) and Huybrecht, Loeckx, Qualyhaegens, DeTobel, and Mistiaen (2011) suggest that mentoring occurs throughout a person's career, and sometime we are the mentor and at other times the mentee. Mentoring occurs at all levels of nursing, is formal or informal, and the mentor can be someone with less experience or education than the mentee if the mentee-mentor relationship allows. There is no one mentoring framework in nursing. There are multiple models that delineate stages of the process for the mentor and mentee. They discuss the importance of nursing students and new graduates learning in classrooms and alongside mentors in clinical practice. They talk about the multiple terms used synonymously with *mentor* such as *preceptor, assessor,* and *supervisor.*

TABLE 2.1
Comparison of Mentoring Roles in the 1990s and 2012

Up to 1995	1995–2012

Role model

No personal relationship need exist. One person internalizes another's behaviors or standards, which then become her or his own (Stewart & Krueger, 1996). Role modeling is considered a way of demonstrating professionalism in nursing by the instructor to the student (Bidwell & Brazier, 1989).

Often, no personal relationship exists. Frequently, nurses have several role models for adapting behaviors and strategies that assist with professional and personal growth. *Shadowing* is synonymous with *role modeling*.

Sponsor

Often money is pledged; a group finds an appropriate reference group for an individual or group of individuals (Stewart & Krueger, 1996).

Term not generally used in short- or long-term nursing relationships. May see this term as a senior person who recommends (sponsors) a less experienced individual for membership in a professional organization.

Preceptor

A pairing of an experienced employee and new employee for purposes of orienting the new employee. This is an assigned pairing for a limited amount of time, generally for 2 to 4 weeks (Stewart & Krueger, 1996).

An experienced staff nurse (Benner, 1984; Benner, Tanner, & Chesla, 2009) is paired with a less experienced nurse, new graduate, or student to orient to a position. Certified nurse practitioners with at least 1 year of experience can precept graduate students studying to become nurse practitioners. The preceptor receives credit for recertification for precepting.

Peer strategizer/co-mentor

People of similar age and experience engage in trading information, guidance, and other assistance to improve at least one of the peer's situations (Stewart & Krueger, 1996).

Peer colleagues network to assist each other. Each individual in the peer network receives beneficial outcomes from this sharing of information and resources.

Coach

A training technique used over an individual's employment span by management and generally on a day-to-day basis (Stewart & Krueger, 1996).

The process of coaching or helping an individual to use his or her maximum potential has become more respected and viewed as very beneficial for employees. It is a common process

Up to 1995	1995–2012
	of mentoring nurse managers and administrators. Also, coaching is a short-term relationship whereby the coachee generally pays the coach to teach a specific skill.
Multiple mentoring	
This allows individuals to network and be mentored by several people simultaneously. There is vertical and horizontal mentoring occurring whereby mentees mentor mentors, and each individual does both roles with multiple people at any one time. This process began to evolve in the 1990s.	This simultaneous mentoring network is extremely common today in nursing academia and service.

There are no standard stages of mentoring in nursing. Kram's (1983) stages of a mentoring relationship are standard in education and are reflected in nursing. Bower (2000) presents a Mentor Relationship Model that has three stages, incorporating Kram's stages (Initiation, Cultivation, Separation, and Redefinition), that are frequently used in nursing:

1. *Selection process.* Generally the mentor chooses the mentee, but there are exceptions when the mentee picks the mentor. Bower feels that due to burnout of nurses, there is more interest in mentoring than ever before. Due to this interest in strengthening the profession, more nurse leaders seem to be mentoring more mentees. During this initial stage of the relationship, it is important for the mentor and mentee to determine if they are compatible, assess their similarities and differences, and determine if they have mutual goals. It is significant that both parties develop trust, and it is fairly easy to see if they are going to be able to work effectively together. Once the selection is made, the following must occur: The mentor agrees to spend a specific amount of time with the mentee, the mentor must be willing to open his or her network of colleagues up to the mentee, the mentor must assess if he or she has the skills to assist the mentee in accomplishing goals, and the mentor must give the mentee access or availability.

2. *Goal-setting phase.* The goals may already be developed by the mentee or the mentee's organization. The mentor may have some guidelines to assist in developing goals, or the two may want to mutually develop the goals. Communication is key for success, and the mentor and mentee must have excellent and frequent communication regarding goal evaluation and progress.

3. *Working phase.* Initially, the mentor sets up activities and work for the mentee to accomplish. Once this is completed, the mentee may suggest certain ideas for the mentor to respond to. This brings the relationship to more of an exchange, and the mentor and mentee become more of a team and work together to accomplish the established goals. It is crucial that both the mentor and mentee feel comfortable in giving each other feedback. If goals continue to be accomplished and the team works successfully together, then the transition step of the working phase will occur. This is the transition of mentee to colleague status.

Another mentoring process that depicts three phases, similar to Bower's and Kram's, is Fox and Shephard (1998). Their phases are: (1) recognition and development, (2) limited independence, and (3) termination and realignment. No stages of preceptorships were identified in the literature. However, if the evaluation aspect of a relationship is formal and determines the mentee's fate in a work setting, then the relationship is a preceptorship, not a mentorship. No specific stages of a coaching relationship were identified either.

Bower (2000) shares examples of her experiences as a mentor and also how she was mentored. Mentoring has been studied in all facets of the profession. It is recommended for use in academia (undergraduate through doctoral levels), clinical settings for all roles (this is generally a preceptorship), political arenas, nursing organizations, and as prenurse matching programs in communities during high school or middle school. Ensher and Murphy (2011), Jonson (2008), and The Harvard Business School (2008) discuss strategies for developing mentees and suggest how to maximize outcomes for the mentor, mentee, and the organization.

Mutually Agreed-On Duration

As mentoring evolves into other forms besides the classic dyad relationship, it becomes more difficult to identify specified periods of time for the relationship. Most feel the classic mentoring relationship exists for at least 5 years, and many say these relationships never really end.

Positive Outcomes Generated for Mentor and Mentee

Mentoring is one of the core competencies that leaders must have (Grossman & Valiga, 2009; Iberre, 2000; Lanser, 2000; Mitchell, 2004; Ross, Wenzel, & Mitlyng, 2002). Mentoring that takes place between an experienced nurse leader and a mentee will generate success for both parties, plus the organization that employs each and the profession of nursing. Outcomes such as improved retention rate of graduate nurses (Almada, Carafoli, Flattery, French, & McNamera, 2004), increased leadership skills for nurses (Grossman, 2009; Nickitas, Keida, Nokes, & Neville, 2004), increased faculty tenure and promotions (Abel, 2004; Snelson et al., 2002), and increased use of resources for academia and health care agencies (Kinnaman & Bleich, 2004) are some of the outcomes produced by having a mentoring culture. Partnering continues to be extremely important for institutions of higher education and health care agencies, in order to accomplish the goals of finding clinical placements and recruiting new graduates; however, even more outcomes from these partnerships have evolved. Achieving Magnet status, research collaboration between academicians and clinicians, cost reduction for both parties, tuition-free courses taught at the health care agency, collaborative grant-writing projects, adjunct teaching positions for clinicians, and sharing of resources are some of the benefits of these practice-education collaborations.

Stewart and Krueger (1996) find in their literature review that outcomes generated by the classic mentor and mentee relationship in the early 1990s included the following:

- Progression of one's career
- Development of new investigators
- Empowerment for mentee
- Increased professional knowledge and practice base
- Generativity for mentor
- Increased numbers of minorities in postbaccalaureate programs
- Institutional staff retention
- Professional socialization

Over the last decade, 2001–2011, the following outcomes of classical mentoring seem apparent, although there are no substantiating data:

- Increased mentoring regarding assisting faculty with developing their research trajectories and obtaining outside funding
- Increased mentoring of nursing faculty and doctoral students regarding research in specific institutions

- Generally increased mentoring for those who are culturally diverse or attempts to provide more role modeling, networking, and shadowing experiences
- Increased partnering between academia and health care agencies for nursing students to work with the agency's experienced nurses
- Increased formal and informal matching of experienced practicing nurses by professional organizations with student nurses and new graduates
- Increased matching of middle and high school students interested in nursing with experienced nurses or a specific group of nurses
- Increased recommendations for use in academia, clinical settings for all roles, political arenas, nursing organizations, and in communities for those in middle or high school who are interested in nursing

Ponti (2009) writes that succession planning, or a deliberative method of developing leaders, must include mentoring. She discusses how to create a succession plan and framework for leadership development. MacPhee, Skelton-Green, Bouthillette, and Suryaprakash (2011) reinforce the importance of empowering individuals either by mentors or through connections via work or personal lives so all can maximize their leadership ability. In her book, *Nurses Taking the Lead* (2000), Bower shares her perception of how having and being a mentor gives one the "skill of gaining recognition, power, and the ability to influence others" (p. 255), which is the outcome nurses are seeking.

Caring, Culturally Competent, and Respectful Environment

Mentors, like preceptors and coaches, can help to provide a safer, less chaotic, and less frantic environment for nurses to deliver the highest quality of care. Dombeck (1999) says, "A mentor relationship is a gift, it is a profound and humbling process. The gift comes from knowing a person and from being given the privilege of watching him/her in the process of professional development" (p. 2). She identifies the mentor's and mentee's promise to share resources and experiences faithfully as the most valuable part of this relationship. This promise is set in the context of a covenant and is dependent on the capacity to listen not only to mentees' questions but to their souls. She feels faculty in a professional school and clinicians in a professional discipline are roles that require ethical commitment to assist inexperienced nurses. Another example of how faculty can assist the nursing profession by doing nursing research, and still achieve other outcomes such as helping undergraduate nursing students gain experience in research and helping the faculty increase their scholarship by achieving a publication and/or professional presentation for their dossier, is discussed (Wheeler, Hardie, Schell, & Plowfield, 2008).

THE MENTORING CULTURE

Stewart and Krueger (1996) conducted a concept analysis of mentoring in nursing and suggest its strongest relationship is as a "teaching–learning process for the socialization of nurse scholars and scientists and the proliferation of a body of professional knowledge" (p. 318). Results of this investigation into the state of classical mentoring in nursing reflect what is happening in academia. Byrne and Keefe (2002) offer an excellent synopsis of the impact of mentoring on nursing research. In fact, research appears to be one of the few area in which long-term mentoring relationships are occurring.

Probably due to the nursing shortage, there is also more interest than ever before in mentoring or guiding students, individuals interested in nursing, and nurses. But what does this mean? Why is it that people are willing to reach out and encourage more individuals to enter the nursing profession? Any nurse would say that it is because nurses are able to make a difference and, if there were to be enough nurses, each nurse could finish the day feeling he or she completed what was planned and made a difference with his or her nursing interventions.

Precepting and coaching are parts of the guidance that a mentee can participate in within their mentorship with other individuals, or can set up as a relationship that is separate from a mentorship. Nurses need to broaden their connections with others so that each nurse is introduced to the multiple benefits of being networked. It would be advantageous to begin getting involved with this mentoring spirit early in one's career. For example, student nurses could be mentees in their initial academic training with a faculty member, clinical nurse, or someone in the university setting, or possibly be mentors for first-year students or someone interested in gaining the kind of experience and knowledge that student mentors can offer. It is known that nurses who have been mentors tend to mentor others (Grossman, 2005; Rosser & Taylor, 2009). Stoddard and Tamasy (2009) have found that individuals who have been successfully mentored are more likely to mentor others when compared to those with little or no mentoring experience.

Nurse clinicians can mentor each other as well as new graduates and students, faculty can mentor graduate students regarding their advanced role and in the area of expanding evidence-based practice, and doctoral students can receive mentoring about their research.

Nurse executives can mentor managers, and managers can mentor staff, and so it goes. Depending on where a nurse is in his or her career, he or she can be a mentor, mentee, or both, and can be in a classic mentoring dyad, a peer network, or multiple mentoring relationships. The majority of nurses think of mentoring as a mechanism for career advancement. Nurses need to think about expanding this view to encompass a broader vision that benefits more than their careers. Mentoring can greatly benefit the profession by expanding nursing knowledge and science. Just as Stewart and Krueger (1996) identified in their concept analysis of mentoring that classic mentoring is "a teaching-learning process for the socialization of nurse scholars and scientists and the proliferation of a body of professional knowledge," other types of mentoring are teaching-learning processes by which nurses can be socialized and add findings from evidence-based practice to the body of professional nursing knowledge. This means that more evidence-based practice and study of how nursing influences patient care needs to be conducted on a daily basis where nurses are practicing.

Clinical nurse specialists and the new clinical nurse leader role may allow a mentoring staff member to expand the nursing science base in everyday work with patients. Just as a bench scientist works in his or her discipline, nurses need to use their patient assignments as a base for their research. Similarly, every staff nurse has a responsibility to assess, plan, implement, and evaluate the highest-quality care for patients. By facilitating a mentoring culture, nurses can work smarter and not harder by using every individual at the work setting in a way that maximizes this person's abilities. An expansive mentoring culture in nursing holds exceptional promise for nurses, the profession, the organizations that employ nurses, and, most significantly, patients. The Nurse Research Internship Program, which exemplifies such a culture, allowed staff nurses to spend 72 paid hours working on their research over 6 months and having mentors available to assist them with their research projects (Clancey, 2009). Having this program available to all staff nurses was very exciting for the staff, who were recognized for their research findings and able to share their new research skills, as well as their findings, with the rest of the staff. If all individuals develop mentoring skills, they can be more effective leaders and have more influence in generating positive outcomes for their organizations (Zachary, 2009).

Indicators of a mentoring culture include

- accountability
- alignment
- demand
- infrastructure

- a common mentoring vocabulary
- multiple venues
- reward
- role modeling
- safety net
- training and education (Zachary, 2005)

Zachary (2005) says that an organization that values mentoring has to accept it within its culture. It cannot be considered an add-on. It must be linked with the organization's values and stated in its mission and philosophy. The infrastructure must be supported by human and financial resources. There must be dedicated time spent on training, mentor coaching, and administration of the mentorship. Nurses who are leaders will be accountable for mentoring those who follow them, and also their peers. They will be reimbursed for their contributions. Mission statements and philosophies for universities and health care agencies encompass values that are congruent with fostering mentoring in their organizations. Organizational structure and the culture of institutions reflect the milieu of the infrastructure. Nurse administrators can role model strategies for staff to best support mentoring in their organizations.

Everyone can visualize a specific department, unit, or even health care agency that was especially welcoming and nurturing at some point in their careers. Likewise, one can appreciate the role models who have assisted in shaping one's career direction and status—the special teacher or staff nurse who took the time to show or explain something just one more time. By promoting more recognition of good experiences and role models, as Hudacek does in her books, *Making a Difference: Stories From the Point of Care* (2005) and *A Daybook for Nurses: Making a Difference Each Day* (2004), a culture of mentoring can advance in nursing. Indeed, the profession can decide to foster mentoring in a more comprehensive fashion by engaging each nurse in coaching, precepting, or mentoring peers and less experienced colleagues. Additionally, more experienced nurses can gain invaluable skills and knowledge regarding informatics from less experienced but tech savvy young nurses. By establishing mentoring teams, nurses can foster more comprehensive networks and develop best practices in mentoring.

MENTORING MODELS IN NURSING

Stewart and Krueger (1996) examined 82 research abstracts and articles written between 1977 and 1994 and found six attributes of mentoring by using concept analysis in interpreting the findings. This collection was a randomly chosen sample from the nursing literature in Canada, the United Kingdom, and the United States. Further reviews of the nursing literature in mentoring support all six of the findings:

1. *Mentoring is a teaching and learning strategy.* Literature to support mentoring as a teaching and learning process is presented, but the authors point out that there is no evidence that mentoring is an effective teaching and learning format, which mentoring process has the largest impact on learning, or a rationale for how mentoring can facilitate a comprehensive body of nursing knowledge. Mentoring is critical in doctoral education if the teaching-learning objectives involving research and grant-writing skills, as well as other professional scholarly activities are to be achieved. Over the past decade, this concept of mentoring has continued to evolve exponentially in doctoral education. Master's and baccalaureate education programs seem to have less mentoring and more coaching and try to have transition experiences for seniors that match them with preceptors, not mentors. Health care agencies foster preceptorship with their experienced employees and new employees. It would be interesting to determine how many of these preceptorships develop into mentorships. Professional organizations recommend that every nurse have a mentor, and some organizations try to match their members with nurses interested in the organization's focus. This is more of a coaching and role modeling process and is aimed more at career growth. It is not clear which part of the mentoring process seems to benefit the mentee's career or the profession the most.

2. *A mentoring relationship has reciprocal roles between the mentor and mentee.* This concept has become more universally accepted for a classically defined mentorship. With the increase in peer and multiple mentoring, it becomes evident that both mentors and mentees benefit from the learning generated from the mentorship.

3. *Mentoring assists in advancement of careers for both the mentor and mentee.* Although the majority of mentoring relationships concentrate on career development, there is a general move toward increasing efforts of mentoring to include development of the profession. Ardery (1990) proposes that mentors and mentees focus on professional success versus personal career success so that knowledge generated from the mentorship can advance nursing theory. This does not seem to have occurred, since research is still dominated by measurements of mentee success with publications, presentations, obtaining grants in their specific area of research, and rate of tenure, promotion, and other gauges of career advancement.

4. *There is generally a knowledge differential between the mentor and mentee.* The idea of the mentor being more knowledgeable than the mentee continues to hold true in classically defined mentoring relationships. However, the growth in the number of peer mentoring and multiple mentoring relationships provides some evidence that this concept may be arguable.
5. *A classic mentorship consists of a long-term relationship extending over several years.* Mentoring relationships on the average tend to endure. This literature review revealed a range of between 1.5 and 33 years.
6. *Mentoring tends to generate resonance.* Mentoring assists participants in developing character and doing higher-quality work.

These six themes seem to be congruent with what is current now, with the added emphasis on mentoring for the profession so nursing can grow. There is also no formal evaluation process in most mentoring relationships unless one counts evaluating the mutually drawn up objectives by the mentor and mentee.

MENTORING IN CLINICAL SETTINGS

There are multiple accounts of supporting new graduates in internships or extended orientations, retooling nurses who have not practiced for a time, and orienting experienced nurses to new experiences (Gilmore, Kopeikin, & Douche, 2007; Scott, 2005). Nurse managers also need to hone their own career guidance skills to effectively develop staff nurses as employees. Help with acclimatizing to a new job and advancing one's career greatly assists a new nurse's successful transition from student to entry-level staff. More generally, mentoring will assist the profession at large within the context of the worldwide nursing shortage by helping to decrease attrition in educational programs while increasing recruitment and retention in health care agencies. In a study by Boswell and Wilhoit (2004), nurses ($N = 67$) identified the following three processes as being what they perceived as most responsible for generating high-quality nursing:

1. Comprehensive orientation on hiring or transfering to a new unit
2. A variety of continuing education programs offered frequently and at the hospital
3. Mentoring

Of course, it is possible that a new graduate will be involved in a preceptorship that will progress to a mentor-mentee relationship. After the new graduate satisfies the competency-based objectives at the end of orientation for his or her unit, the preceptor and the new graduate may wish to extend their relationship on a more informal and non-evaluative basis. The relationship could then become a mentorship. Often, new graduates or any nurses transitioning to a specialty unit develop a peer mentoring network that is extremely helpful in their transition to staff nurse status (Grossman, 2011).

It is important to realize that the relationship or mentorship will extend beyond the specific job and assist the new nurse in becoming socialized into the professional nurse's role.

Angelini (1995) conducted a qualitative grounded theory study to identify how mentoring influenced the career development of hospital staff nurses. Environment, people, and events were identified as significant to mentoring. Both the staff nurses and manager defined mentoring as broader than just the dyad. The nurses felt that the environment consisted of what the hospital offered them, such as tuition reimbursement, other educational opportunities at the hospital, chances to consult with other nurses, and financial rewards. "People" included both primary and secondary mentors (people who influenced them), with the primary ones being nurse managers and peer staff nurses with whom they interacted frequently and the secondary people being less frequent contacts, such as clinical nurse specialists, nurse educators, family members, and physicians. "Events" included occurrences perceived to be critical to career development, such as clinical patient situations and career incidents (first job, first charge, first transfer, first float). And outside influences involved family, social events, and issues such as the women's movement. Angelini's conclusions include that true mentoring takes on primary importance at the clinical bedside but generally does occur in every aspect of life.

There are studies of students doing their capstone experience, often in their senior year, who have had a semester-long, assigned "mentor"—literally, a preceptor. Each preceptorship is different and is influenced by multiple variables. Some (Greene & Puetzer, 2002; Grossman, 2005) suggest that the prime time to introduce nurses to a mentor relationship is during the student experience since academia is responsible for preparing nurses for their first roles, in patient care delivery. Several have published their experiences in providing students with some form of mentoring in a nursing care setting. Grossman (2005) describes a shadowing experience for senior students in a leadership and management rotation in which each student was assigned a leader in a health care agency to shadow over a semester. Findings revealed statistically significant increased leadership development scores after the mentorship. Papp, Markkanen, and von Bonsdorff (2003) reported that student nurses perceived more positive learning environments when nurse educators and staff nurses worked closely together in providing precepted clinical experiences.

In the United Kingdom, practice learning accounts for nearly 50% of the prequalifying nursing program. Andrews and Wallis (1999) thus were most interested in determining what teaching-learning strategies best support students. They found that mentorship is widely relied on to teach the main activities associated with practice skills. Nurse educators in the United Kingdom also use the mentorship strategy in classroom and clinical teaching.

In Australia, The Institute of Nursing Executives responded to concerns expressed by their membership regarding nurse managers who work in rural areas by developing a mentoring program to provide professional development and support networks for such nurses. A pilot program that ran in and around Sydney required managers and mentors to attend a full-day mentoring workshop. There was time set aside for mentors and mentees to form partnerships. Seventy-nine percent of the participants responded to a preworkshop questionnaire asking for their most significant learning needs. They cited learning how to increase their confidence in coaching and stimulating staff as their primary learning need. Managers' evaluations of the program expressed a need for more networking, more structured mentoring, and training to assist them in using technology to keep involved in their newly established mentorships and networks. Outcomes of the project included the development of a mentoring listserv and website to assist managers (Waters, Clarke, Ingall, & Dean-Jones, 2003).

There are also studies of graduate students being precepted. Research indicates a definitive need for these programs to retain nurses and prepare them adequately for RN, APRN, and DNP positions. Hayes (1998, 2001) discusses factors that increase self-efficacy as well as mentoring scores for nurse practitioner students and points out that nurse practitioner students do better with self-efficacy scores if they can pick their own mentor nurse practitioner, particularly if they had a previous relationship with that person. This information is especially helpful for nurse practitioner program directors who may have been making extremely time-consuming assignments of procuring preceptors. Also, it is necessary to mentor or precept nurse practitioner students regarding other activities that affect patient care but are not involved in direct care, such as research, consultation, counseling, teaching, quality assurance, case management, and health policy development. Hawkins and Fontenot (2009) emphasize the importance of mentoring nurse practitioner students in all aspects of the role since their primary precepting involves the clinical practice focus. It is, therefore, extremely important for nurse practitioner faculty to role model and provide seminars, share relevant experiences about their own practice, and provide opportunities for their students during the educational period. Often, graduate nurse practitioners keep in touch with their teachers for advice on negotiating contracts, obtaining malpractice insurance and affiliation privileges, and just talking about day-to-day practice concerns. Additionally, junior nurse practitioner faculty need careful mentoring regarding setting up rotations and insuring that the students are adequately taught the complete role of the nurse practitioner. The National Organization of Nurse Practitioner Faculty (NONPF) has a website, www.nonpf.org, with resources for mentoring nurse practitioner students as well as graduates.

Due to low staffing, heavy acuity, and lack of resources, there is an intense need for appropriate supervision and mentorship of nursing students. The School of Nursing at the University of Nottingham, England, developed a student peer support supervision program in which senior students supervise and support junior students in their clinical rotations under the mentorship of a clinical nurse. Three themes were identified after analyzing results of a questionnaire given to 31 seniors and 27 juniors:

- Preparation for clinical assignment
- Support and feedback regarding their performance
- Personal and professional development

This program was evaluated overwhelmingly positively by both groups of students. Seniors commented on improving their teaching and mentoring skills, and juniors felt the program helped to decrease their anxiety and provide needed support (Aston & Molassiotis, 2003).

MENTORING AND CLASSROOM TEACHING

Andrews and Roberts (2003) say mentoring is important in the classroom as well as in clinical rotations. Nurse educators need to mentor their students. Nurse educators can assist students to be academically successful. Gilmore, Kopeikin, and Douche (2007) found a significant relationship between faculty support and student retention and success. It is evident that undergraduate faculty will not be able to have a classic mentoring relationship with every student. Rather, faculty can mentor in groups, assist students in finding preceptors in their clinical rotations, and advise students in groups as well as individually as situations arise and also in anticipation of specific events. Graduate faculty need to mentor their students in the more traditional way or find a preceptor who will be working with the graduate student and could serve as a mentor. Doctoral students should have a classic mentor in order to be successful with their research. Nursing faculty engaged in research are the best mentors for students. These students need to develop grantsmanship and research skills, and become connected to the other researchers in their chosen area of study (Byrne & Keefe, 2002). Faculty mentors must assist with increasing self-esteem, be available for support and advice, be a good role model by teaching by example, try to connect students to opportunities for new experiences, try to support passion and vision, and give career advice.

After graduation, most new graduates are assigned to a preceptor, and if they have had experience with some form of mentoring, they will most likely maximize their experience as a preceptee (Jokelainen, Turunen, Tossavainen, Jamookeeah, & Coco, 2011). The preceptee will also know the advantages of trying to continue a supportive relationship with the preceptor after orientation ends. Simultaneously, new graduates will be aware of the advantages of keeping their relationship with someone from their school of nursing or will begin to shape a new relationship with someone at their employing agency. New graduates can foster the mentoring culture in their work settings by demonstrating behavior that recognizes the importance of encouraging and supporting others.

Multiple mentoring encourages maximal growth and probably increases outcomes at the work or school setting. This win-win combination is the future of a more collaborative working nurse force. Turning from a task orientation to more of a relationship paradigm will allow for improved work production and assist the nurse in delegating and seeing patients differently.

There have been several courses offered for undergraduate nursing students that involved long-term mentoring after the official completion of the semester or mentorships for new orienting nurses that have continued after the orientation (Jakubik, 2008; Morrison-Beady, Aronowitz, Dyne, & Mkandawire, 2001). Byrne and Keefe (2002) recommend that more mentoring in research be performed with undergraduate and master's students. They believe that more mentored research will occur where there are more faculty funded by the National Institutes of Health

(NIH) and other funding agencies who need research assistants and at universities with academic health centers conducting clinical research.

MENTORING DOCTORAL STUDENTS

Byrne and Keefe (2002) relate that one of the major foci of classic mentoring in nursing has shifted to mentoring nurse researchers. They provide descriptions of strategies for setting up research mentorships and describe five research mentoring models:

- Traditional one-on-one mentor to mentee
- A team of mentors working with one mentee
- Peer-to-peer mentors
- One mentor and a group of mentees
- Initial traditional mentor to mentee, which then becomes a collegial peer relationship

There is a critical need for development of nurse researchers and only a limited number of institutions are equipped to prepare scholars in an accelerated manner. Providing mentoring throughout undergraduate and graduate education by funded faculty researchers is advocated. Accelerated NIH-funded schools with research-intensive tracks that link baccalaureate through doctoral education right to postdoctoral training are needed in order to prepare nurse research academicians. Perhaps a program similar to the 7-year premedical and medical school programs could be a model for nurses to build a similar prenursing and nurse doctoral program. Faculty at the University of Northern Colorado developed a PhD nursing program online and their first-year outcomes show positive evaluation by students regarding the mentoring they received from faculty, the amount of time they had faculty interaction, and the socialization to the doctoral program they felt they achieved (Leners, Wilson, & Sitzman, 2007).

MENTORING OF FACULTY

Records and Emerson (2003) share a comprehensive research skill development mentoring model they developed for new faculty at their institution that includes assigning the mentee to two seasoned faculty researchers. The researchers assist in developing annual goals over a 6-year time span, such as submitting two manuscripts, presenting at one conference, and obtaining at least one potential consultant who can assist them with their research funding the first year. The mentors schedule meetings along the 6-year time line. Mentors read the new faculty member's dissertation and assist the person in developing manuscript ideas, select the top researchers in the mentee's field who are in the geographical area, assist with grant writing, suggest methods for networking with them and ways to access research participants and funding, and even give advice concerning how to gracefully decline offers of assistance from those who do not facilitate progress. With the nursing faculty shortage, it would seem prudent for all schools of nursing to engage in a similar mentoring program for new faculty.

Byrne and Keefe (2002) reviewed the literature on research mentoring of faculty. They describe one study of 305 doctorally prepared female faculty working in graduate programs in the United States. Only 56% of the participants reported having had mentorships; however, having a mentorship did not correlate highly with funded research. The actual productivity of scholarship was higher for both the mentee and mentor than for faculty who were not in a mentorship. Targeted mentoring relationships were started at the University of Louisville, which connected faculty with productive researchers outside the institution (Mundt, 2001). This strategy did result in increased productivity and funding. Carlson and Rotondo (2001) cite that tenured full professors who are committed to succession planning for the profession are able to do the most mentoring. If they are not involved in funded research, they will be unable to properly mentor new faculty with their scholarship needs. This is where the nonfunded research faculty could mentor the junior faculty for service and teaching but acquire assistance from outside the institution for research mentoring.

Gray and Armstrong (2003) cite the need for new training and nurturing of young research faculty and especially target the need for nurse researchers. They offer suggestions for developing new programs to train and mentor a critical mass of nurse academics so they will be able to assume leadership. They recommend the Quebec Model of Support Health Research Networks, which fosters more cross-discipline training and mentoring of nurses and other members of the health team.

INTERNATIONAL MENTORING

Byrne and Keefe (2002) report on the multiple partnerships that are occurring across boundaries regarding common patient care issues. There is much disparity between the programs regarding resources for research, so there has emerged a great need for mentoring. With today's technology, mentors can communicate with mentees or coach a group of faculty in another country easily. The classic mentoring method does not tend to be successful due to the distance and multiple needs of many of the mentees. The multiple mentoring and peer mentoring models seem as if they will be most effective. There is an abundance of advantages from mentoring and conducting international research (Braitwaite, 2002). An effective mentoring model that provides international and interdisciplinary scholars in grounded theory to mentor doctoral students in all areas of the world is described by Nathaniel (2009).

CULTURALLY COMPETENT MENTORING

Martin, Yarbrough, and Alfred (2003) conducted a study of associate and baccalaureate nursing degree graduates in Texas ($N = 1,450$) with the Nurses Professional Value Scale (NPVS) to measure their professional values. Their findings revealed no difference in total score; however, the associate degree graduates did significantly better than baccalaureate graduates on five of the scales: client privacy, accountability for nursing action, acceptance of responsibility and seeks consultation when appropriate, participation in efforts to improve standards of nursing, and collaboration with other team members to meet health needs of public. Their findings suggest the need for increased mentoring regarding professional values, especially with diverse student populations.

The fact that there is a separate component of this chapter on multicultural competence speaks to the lack of integration of cultural competency in the many mentoring models. Most preceptors are not of the same culture as their preceptee, so it is of utmost importance to have preceptors trained in cultural competency. Actually, all nurses and health care workers should be trained, and there should be multiple strategies by which heightened awareness and linkage to academic success could be achieved (Valencia, 2005).

For example, Wilson, Sanner, and McAllister (2010) performed focus groups with 10 faculty and 30 junior and senior nursing student mentees and determined their perceptions of how the mentorship had succeeded. The faculty felt their role modeling and caring had greatly impacted the mentees' success with course grades as well as their NCLEX scores. Students found the faculty to be an excellent support that assisted them with their course grades and NCLEX scores and also increased their perceptions of what the nursing profession offered them as a career. Some mentors and mentees may be from the same culture but have very different levels of cultural sensitivity. Coffman, Shellman, and Bernal (2004) suggest that nurses lack cultural self-efficacy, information, and experience with culturally diverse groups. Cultural stereotypes for Asian Americans, Hispanic Americans, and African Americans need to be dispersed, and perhaps doing role plays of some of these issues would serve to increase awareness among preceptors so they do not show prejudice to their preceptees and the preceptees do not stereotype their preceptors.

EXAMPLES OF DEVELOPING MENTORING IN NURSING

Mentoring has become so important that the American Nurses Association (ANA) sent out a call for proposals for mentoring programs for nurses in 2011. Five of the state associations who submitted proposals were selected for funding by the ANA and are now implementing their programs in their states (American Nurses Association [ANA], 2011). The taskforce for this mentoring project defined mentoring as: "A one-to-one trusting relationship that encompasses formal or informal supporting, guiding, coaching, teaching, role modeling, counseling, advocating and networking. Mentoring occurs within and/or outside the clinical setting and includes personal and career guidance. Mentoring promotes co-sharing, co-discovery, and co-growth" (ANA, 2011, p. 1). Their purpose of the mentoring programs is "to support the growth and development of nurses as they transition in professional practice; to foster the development of a strong nursing community; and to enhance the leadership skills of nurses as they engage in the mentoring process" (ANA, 2011, p. 1).

Sigma Theta Tau International has several mentoring programs offered through their Leadership Institute including the Mentored Leadership Program, Board Leadership Development Program, Maternal Child Health Leadership Academy, Nurse Faculty Mentored Leadership Development Program, and Geriatric Nursing Leadership Academy, which can all be located on the organization's website, www.nursingsociety.org. The list goes on and on, so no nurse can honestly say there are not resources to access for connecting with mentoring programs either as a mentor or mentee. Finally, the Center for Creative Leadership (CCL) has a program, *Developing the Leader*, which has excellent ideas on how to mentor and maximize the benefits of a mentoring relationship. They ascribe to working on guiding one's professional development, the team members one works with, and one's organization in order to increase everyone's creative leadership and success (Center for Creative Leadership [CCL], 2011). Additionally, the Center for Creative Leadership has published a book, *Seven Keys to Effective Mentoring* (2009), authored by Hart, that outlines ideas for developing a mentoring program for whatever your organization's needs are (CCL, 2011) and CLL also has an online *Mentoring Guide* (2003). The National Mentoring Network (2012) based in the United Kingdom, which can be accessed at www.mentors.ca, provides information on mentoring definitions, gender issues in mentoring, mentoring as a driver for change, finding a mentor, developing a mentor and mentee contract, and evaluating mentoring. The Oncology Nursing Society (2009) has multiple mentoring programs such as Advocacy Mentoring, Mentor/Fellow Writing, Ethnic Minority Mentoring, Abstract Writers Mentoring, Member-to-Member Mentorimg, Student Mentoring, and Leader Consultation Pool programs.

Just about every professional journal publishes several articles a year on mentoring. Table 2.2 indicates some selected examples for the year 2011. Since the mid-1990s, there have been articles explaining mentoring programs with RNs or nursing students being paired with a more experienced person to achieve a specific goal—usually to orient or educate the less experienced person to a new position or, in some instances, to the profession of nursing. What generally is not as clear is what the authors mean by mentoring. Most of the articles listed in Table 2.2 identify role modeling/shadowing, precepting, and coaching

TABLE 2.2
Selected Examples of Mentoring Articles, 2011

Journal and Author	Article Title
International Nursing Review (Li, H.-C., Wang, L. S., Lin, Y.-H., & Lee, I., 2011)	"The effect of a peer-mentoring strategy on student nurse stress reduction in clinical practice"
Nursing 2011 Critical Care (Grossman, S., 2011)	"Using collaborative mentoring in critical care"
Journal of Professional Nursing (Gwyn, P. G., 2011)	"The quality of mentoring relationships' impact on the occupational commitment of nursing faculty"
Nurse Education Today (Siu, G. P., & Sivan, A., 2011)	"Mentoring experiences of psychiatric nurses: From acquaintance to affirmation"
Nursing Education Perspectives (Cottingham, S., DiBartolo, M. C., Battistoni, S., & Brown, T., 2011)	"Partners in nursing: A mentoring initiative to enhance nurse retention"
Nurse Educator (Harmer, B. M., Huffman, J., & Johnson, B., 2011)	"Clinical peer mentoring"

rather than the classic mentoring relationship even though they use the term *mentor* in their title.

It would seem that just about any contact one can have from an experienced individual is a positive experience for the nurse or student. These accounts will assist in developing a mentoring culture in the profession. Likewise, it seems that most mentors benefit from being a mentor (Huybrecht et al., 2011; Liu, Liu, Kwan, & Mao, 2009). Observing nurse leaders helps new nurses cultivate new skills in leadership, management, and clinical practice.

CONCLUSION

There is the beginning of a mentoring culture in the nursing profession, as evidenced by accounts in the literature of successful mentoring in the clinical arena with nurses, advanced practice nurses, managers, and students, as well as in the classroom. Mentoring is evolving to more of a multiple mentor process for most nurses except for doctoral students and junior faculty. It is paramount that nurses use best practices in mentoring regarding the various components of the process:

- A guided but nonevaluated experience
- Formal versus informal assignment/stages of relationship
- Mutually agreed-on duration
- Positive outcomes generated (this includes reciprocity) for mentor and mentee
- Caring, culturally competent, respectful environment

There is more awareness of the need for continued mentoring with international research initiatives as well. Benefits from these partnerships will gain recognition for the mentor, mentee, the involved organizations, and the profession.

Mentoring in nursing encompasses a guided experience, whether it is formally or informally assigned over a mutually agreed-on period that empowers the mentor and mentee to develop personally and professionally within the auspices of a caring, collaborative, culturally competent, and respectful environment. Evidence-based practice in mentoring in nursing can support each component of this definition.

REFERENCES

Abel, E. (2004). Faculty response to faculty-nurse mentoring. *Journal of Holistic Nursing, 22,* 186–188.

Almada, P., Carafoli, K., Flattery, J., French, D., & McNamera, M. (2004). Improving the retention rate of newly graduated nurses. *Journal for Nurses in Staff Development, 20,* 268–273.

American Nurses Association. (2011). *Mentoring programs for nurses.* ANA Request for Proposals. Retrieved from http://nursingworld.org/DocumentVault/NewsAnnouncements/ANA-Demonstration-Mentoring-Program-Memo.pdf., p. 1

Andrews, M., & Roberts, D. (2003). Supporting student nurses learning in and through clinical practice: The role of the clinical guide. *Nurse Education Today, 23,* 474–481.

Andrews, M., & Wallis, M. (1999). Mentorship in nursing: A literature review. *Journal of Advanced Nursing, 29,* 201–207.

Angelini, D. (1995). Mentoring in the career development of hospital staff nurses: Models and strategies. *Journal of Professional Nursing, 11,* 89–97.

Ardery, G. (1990). Mentors and protégés: From ideology to knowledge. In J. McCloskey & H. Grace (Eds.), *Current issues in nursing* (pp. 58–63). St. Louis, MO: Mosby.

Aston, L., & Molassiotis, A. (2003). Supervising and supporting student nurses in clinical placements: The peer support initiative. *Nurse Education Today, 23,* 202–210.

Benner, P. (1984). *From novice to expert: Excellence and power in clinical nursing practice.* Menlo Park, CA: Addison-Wesley.

Benner, P., Tanner, C., & Chesla, C. (2009). *Expertise in nursing practice: Caring, clinical judgment, and ethics.* New York, NY: Springer.

Bidwell, A. S., & Brasier, M. L. (1989). Role modeling versus mentoring in nursing education. *Journal of Nursing Scholarship, 21*(1), 23–25.

Boswell, S., & Wilhoit, K. (2004). New nurses' perceptions of nursing practice and quality patient care. *Journal of Nursing Care Quality, 19,* 76–81.

Bower, F. (2000). *Nurses taking the lead: Personal qualities of effective leadership.* Philadelphia, PA: Saunders.

Braitwaite, D. (2002). Mentoring relationships while conducting international research. *Multicultural Nursing Health, 8,* 36–41.

Byrne, M., & Keefe, M. (2002). Building research competence in nursing through mentoring. *Journal of Nursing Scholarship, 34,* 391–396.

Carlson, D., & Rotondo, C. (2001). Building research competence in nursing through mentoring. *Advanced Nursing, 27,* 1296–1304.

Center for Creative Leadership. (2003). *Mentoring guide: A guide for mentors.* Retrieved from http://www.cfhl.org/FileServlet2?id=7

Center for Creative Leadership. (2011). *Center for creative leadership.* Retrieved from http://www.ccl.org/leadership/about/index.aspx

Clancey, J. K.(2009). Nursing research internship program: A unique mentoring program. *Journal of Neuroscience Nursing, 41*(6), E1–E6.

Coffman, M., Shellman, J., & Bernal, H. (2004). An integrative review of American nurses' perceived cultural self-efficacy. *Journal of Nursing Scholarship, 36,* 180–185.

Cottingham, S., DiBartolo, M. C., Battistoni, S., & Brown, T., 2011. Partners in nursing: A mentoring initiative to enhance nurse retention. *Nursing Education Perspectives, 32(4), 250–255.*

Dombeck, M. (1999). The mentor relationship. *Research in Nursing and Health, 22,* 1–2.

Ensher, E. A., & Murphy, S. E. (2011). *Power mentoring: How successful mentors and protégés get the most out of their relationships.* San Francisco, CA: Jossey-Bass.

Fox, S., & Shephard, T. (1998). The essence of mentoring. *Journal of Neuroscience Nursing, 30,* 1–3.

Gilmore, J. A., Kopeiken, A., & Douche, J. (2007). Student nurses as peer mentors: Collegiality in practice. *Nurse Education in Practice, 7(1),* 36–43.

Gray, J., & Armstrong, P. (2003). Academic health leadership: Looking to the future. *Clinical Investigational Medicine, 26,* 315–326.

Greene, M., & Puetzer, M. (2002). The value of mentoring: A strategic approach to retention and recruitment. *Journal of Nursing Care Quality, 17,* 63–70.

Grossman, S. (2005). Developing leadership through shadowing a leader in health care. In H. Feldman & M. Greenberg (Eds.), *Educating for leadership* (Ch. 25, pp. 266–278). New York, NY: Springer.

Grossman, S. (2011). Using collaborative mentoring in critical care. *Nursing 2011 Critical Care, 6(3),* 38–41.

Grossman, S., & Valiga, T. (2009). *The new leadership challenge: Creating the future of nursing* (3rd ed.). Philadelphia, PA: F. A. Davis.

Gwyn, P. G., (2011). The quality of mentoring relationships' impact on the occupational commitment of nursing faculty. *Journal of Professional Nursing, 27(5),* 292–298.

Harmer, B. M., Huffman, J., & Johnson, B., (2011). Clinical peer mentoring. *Nurse Educator, 36(5),* 197–202.

Hart, E. W. (2009). *Seven keys to successful mentoring.* Oakland, CA: Center for Creative Leadership Press.

The Harvard Business School. (2008). *Coaching and mentoring: How to develop top talent and achieve stronger performance.* Cambridge, MA: Harvard Business School Press.

Hawkins, J. W., & Fontenot, H. (2009). What do you mean you want me to teach, do research, engage in service, and clinical practice? Views from the trenches: The novice, the expert. *Journal of American Academy of Nurse Practitioners, 21(7),* 358–361.

Hayes, E. (1998). Mentoring and nurse practitioner student self-efficacy. *Western Journal of Nursing Research, 20,* 521–535.

Hayes, E. (2001). Factors that facilitate or hinder mentoring in the nurse practitioner preceptor/student relationship. *Clinical Excellence for Nurse Practitioners, 5,* 111–118.

Hudacek, S. (2004). *A daybook for nurses: Making a difference each day.* Indianapolis, IN: Center Nursing Press.

Hudacek, S. (Ed.). (2005). *Making a difference: Stories from the point of care.* Indianapolis, IN: Sigma Theta Tau International.

Huybrecht, S., Loeckx, W., Quaeyhaegens, Y., DeTobel, D., & Mistiaen, W. (2011). Mentoring in nursing education: Perceived characteristics of mentors and the consequences of mentorship. *Nursing Education Today, 31*(3), 274–278.

Iberre, H. (2000). Making partner: A mentor's guide to the psychological journey. *Harvard Business Review, 78,* 148–149.

Jakubik, L. D. (2008). Mentoring beyond the first year: Predictors of mentoring benefits for pediatric staff nurse protégés. *Journal of Pediatric Nursing, 23*(4), 269–281.

Jokelainen, M., Turunen, H., Tossavainen, K., Jamookeeah, D., & Coco, K. (2011). A systematic review of mentoring nursing students in clinical placements. *Journal of Clinical Nursing, 20*(19/20), 2854–2867.

Jonson, K. F. (2008). *Being an effective mentor: How to help beginning teachers succeed* (2nd ed.). Thousand Oaks, CA: Corwin Press.

Kinnaman, M., & Bleich, M. (2004). Collaboration: Aligning resources to create and sustain partnerships. *Journal of Professional Nursing, 20,* 310–322.

Kram, K. (1983). Phases of the mentor relationship. *Academy of Management Journal, 26,* 608–625.

Lanser, E. (2000). Reaping the benefits of mentorship. *Healthcare Executive, 15,* 19–23.

Leners, D. W., Wilson, V. W., & Sitzman, K. L. (2007). Twenty-first century doctoral education: Online with a focus on nursing education. *Nursing Education Perspectives, 28*(6), 332–336.

Li, H.-C., Wang, L. S., Lin, Y.-H., & Lee, I. (2011). The effect of a peer-mentoring strategy on student nurse stress reduction in clinical practice. *International Nursing Review, 58*(2), 203–210.

Liu, D., Liu, J., Kwan, H. K., & Mao, Y. (2009). What can I gain as a mentor? The effect of mentoring on the job performance and social status of mentors in China. *Journal of Occupational and Organizational Psychology, 82* (Pt. 4), 871–895.

MacPhee, M., Skelton-Green, J., Bouthillette, F., & Suryaprakash, N. (2011). An empowerment framework for nursing leadership development: Supporting evidence. *Journal of Advanced Nursing, 68*(1), 159–169.

Martin, P., Yarbrough, S., & Alfred, D. (2003). Professional values held by baccalaureate and associate degree nursing students. *Journal of Nursing Scholarship, 35,* 291–296.

Mitchell, G. (2004). The mentoring of nurses: Possibilities for times of transition. *Nursing Science Quarterly, 17,* 317–324.

Morrison-Beady, D., Aronowitz, T., Dyne, J., & Mkandawire, L. (2001). Mentoring students and junior faculty in funded research: A win-win scenario. *Journal of Professional Nursing, 17,* 291–296.

Mundt, M. H. (2001). An external mentor program: Stimulus for faculty research development. *Journal of Professional Nursing, 17,* 40–45.

Nathaniel, A. K. (2009, March 1). A model for international, interdisciplinary research mentoring: 2009 Southern nursing research society conference. *Southern Online Journal of Nursing Research, 9*(2), 1.

National Mentoring Network. (2012). *Peer resources.* Retrieved from http://www.mentors.ca/

Nickitas, D., Keida, R., Nokes, K., & Neville, S. (2004). Nurturing nursing future through nurse executive partnerships. *Nursing Economics, 22,* 258–263.

Oncology Nursing Society. (2009). ONS mentoring programs provide learning and networking opportunities. *ONS Connect, 1,* 26.

Papp, T., Markkanen, M., & von Bonsdorff, M. (2003). Clinical environment as a learning environment: Student nurses' perceptions concerning clinical learning experiences. *Nurse Education Today, 23,* 262–268.

Ponti, M. (2009). Transition from leadership development to succession management. *Nursing Administration Quarterly, 33*(2), 125–141.

Records, K., & Emerson, R. (2003). Mentoring for research skill development. *Journal of Nursing Education, 42,* 553–557.

Restifo, V., & Yoder, L. (2004). Partnership: Making the most of mentoring. *Nursing Spectrum, 8,* 16–19.

Ross, A., Wenzel, F., & Mitlyng, J. (2002). *Leadership for the future: Core competencies in health care.* Chicago, IL: Health Administration Press.

Rosser, S., & Taylor, Z. (2009). Why are we still worried about women in science? *Academe Bulletin of the AAUP, 95*(3), 6–10.

Scott, E. S. (2005). Peer-to peer mentoring: Teaching collegiality. *Nurse Educator, 30,* 52–56.

Siu, G. P., & Sivan, A. (2011). Mentoring experiences of psychiatric nurses: From acquaintance to affirmation. *Nurse Education Today, 31*(8), 797–802.

Snelson, C., Martsolf, D., Dieckman, B., Anaya, E., Cartehine, K., Miller, B., & Shaffer, J. (2002). Caring as a theoretical perspective for a nursing faulty mentoring program: Mentoring program for new faculty. *Nursing Education Today, 22,* 654–660.

Stewart, B., & Krueger, L. (1996). An evolutionary concept analysis of mentoring in nursing. *Journal of Professional Nursing, 12,* 311–321.

Stoddard, D. A., & Tamasy, R. J. (2009). *The heart of mentoring: 10 proven principles.* Colorado Springs, CO: NAVPRESS.

Valencia-Go, G. (2005). Growth and access increase for nursing students: A retention and progression project. *Journal of Cultural Diversity, 12*(1), 18–25.

Waters, D., Clarke, M., Ingall, A., & Dean-Jones, M. (2003). Evaluation of a pilot mentoring program for nurse managers. *Journal of Advanced Nursing, 42,* 516–526.

Wheeler, E. C., Hardie, T., Schell, K., & Plowfield, L. (2008). Symbiosis—undergraduate research mentoring and faculty scholarship in nursing. *Nursing Outlook, 56*(1), 9–15.

Wilson, A. H., Sanner, S. & McAllister, L. E. (2010). An evaluation of a student mentoring program to increase the diversity of the nursing workforce. *Journal of Cultural Diversity, 17*(4), 144–150.

Zachary, L. (2005). *Creating a mentoring culture: The organization's guide.* San Francisco, CA: Jossey-Bass.

Zachary, L. (2009). *The mentee's guide: Making mentoring work for you.* San Francisco, CA: Jossey-Bass.

3

Coaching Each Other to Empower

One way leaders empower and assist others to empower themselves is by respecting each person and the person's ability to contribute to an organization and the profession. Certain variables such as organizational culture, the leadership style of the nurse and other administrators, and the current collaborative practice or faculty governance model have an impact on how empowered nurses can be in their work setting. Due to the high patient acuity and demand for nurses and the scarce resources in both practice and academia, the environment is ripe for nurse leaders to think creatively about new ways to accomplish work. In this way, they can use their leadership ability in empowering others to capture what they want to do to make a difference in their everyday work, their career path, and for the nursing profession. It is necessary for nurses to increase their autonomy in the clinical arena, gain momentum in carving out areas of research that will strengthen nursing science, add to evidence-based practice, and network together to create partnerships to fulfill both clinical and academic missions. This chapter thus describes the concept of empowerment; strategies to help empower oneself, others, and the profession; a comparison of empowerment with the enabling process; and how creating a mentoring culture will empower the profession.

EMPOWERMENT

Empowerment means being inspired with self-confidence and the knowledge that one can make a difference by one's actions. It eventually leads to increased self-esteem. *Empowering*, or being able to empower others, is defined as being able to encourage an individual or oneself with confidence and demonstrating the ability to exude a sense of authority to another person or oneself. It is exactly what nurses need rather than being enabled to fulfill orders from members of other disciplines. The hierarchical structure that has existed for decades is changing, and staff nurses, advanced practice nurses, and nurse administrators are assuming more equitable positions of authority. Wheatley (2006), in explaining the new science of leadership, recommends empowering all and decreasing the constraints of bureaucratic structures in order to improve productivity and quality. This paradigm change supports people in achieving higher self-esteem as an outcome of feeling more self-confident in their work settings. Supportive evidence of this statement is the empowerment framework for nursing leadership development used with mid-level nurse leaders in one health care organization (MacPhee, Skelton-Green, Bouthillette, & Suryaprakash, 2011).

To improve understanding, however, one should be able to differentiate between self-confidence and self-esteem. Self-confidence encompasses how an individual feels at a given time and can be affected by many variables, such as one's health or even the weather. Self-esteem is a constant feeling of acceptance for the person one is. It is not influenced by everyday events. It is a way of being.

Certain steps need to occur before an individual nurse or a unit's staff can become empowered. For example, imagine an orthopedic unit where the surgeons never communicate with the nursing staff and continue to send them unstable postoperative patients and multiple admissions without bothering to develop any clinical protocols to follow. The surgeons and technicians treat the nurses without respect and recognition for their work. If the attitude were to change in a setting like this, nurses would have to be able to recognize the negative atmosphere they were working in and, at the same time, be aware that this type of demeaning, or poor work environment was not present on other nursing units. Second, the nurses would need to be extremely competent with their knowledge and expertise in their clinical specialties, as well as have effective communication skills to support their self-esteem. Finally, the staff would have to be resourceful enough to be able to negotiate with the administration, and allow them to engage physicians toward creating a new work atmosphere.

Empowerment of an organization's workers is considered one of the most important aspects of whether or not an organization achieves excellence (Grossman & Valiga, 2009). All individuals need to feel successful and self-directed in order to generate excellence and accomplish the organization's goals. Katzenbach and Khan (2010) offer several good strategies on how to mobilize and energize one's team by using both informal and formal lines to achieve high levels of performance. They also have an *Organizational Quotient Tool* that can help in assessing an organization's ability to use both informal and formal lines.

Nurses need to be recognized for the small wins that staff members achieve every day. This would serve to encourage the profession and give nurses hope that things can change. The unit or department also needs to get away from the idea that perfection is the goal or that nothing is ever good enough. So instead of always accentuating the negative, it is wise to focus on a more positive overall stance. Perhaps then staff will begin to think, act, and behave like winners.

Nurses need to be empowered themselves so that they can help their patients by empowering them to feel they can speak up about their condition and plan of care. Kodish et al. (2004) have found that, when researchers talk with families in clinical trials who have children with leukemia, it helps to have a nurse on hand to reinforce the information and explain and answer questions. These researchers believe that having a nurse available "may reflect the benefits of better emotional support for parents at a difficult time," enabling them to speak up, ask questions, and seek clarification about their children. Empowering patients and their families is a high-level leadership skill that nurses who are self-empowered can do successfully.

Surely times have changed, and nurses today portray a much different image than when "nurses felt rooted in a calling of devotional service and self-sacrificial love, now seen as either repressed middle class women with psychological complexes or women held down as handmaidens of the patriarchal medical establishment" (Bradshaw, 1995, p. 472). Fortunately, empowered nursing leaders have emerged and transformed the profession to seek evidence-based knowledge that is now driving clinical practice, education, and nursing research. This new nursing practice defies the historical roots of the profession's actions and propels nursing toward a better future (Roberts & Vasquez, 2004). A helpful guide, *The Empowerment Manual* by Starhawk (2011), can assist individuals interested in learning new strategies to empower themselves and others.

Kouzes and Posner (2007) describe five sets of behavioral practices that have assisted leaders to become empowered and able to encourage people to do extraordinary things:

- Demonstrate perseverance
- Have a focus or direction
- Empower others
- Be a role model
- Recognize others' contributions

Leadership is a skill that can be developed by coaching and through experiential learning. Kouzes and Posner remind us that leadership is everyone's business, and therefore everyone should accept the leadership challenge on a daily basis. Gershon and Straub (2011) also believe that each individual should empower themselves by seeking their own way to the truth, and following one's vision so that they live to maximize their potential.

In her 2003 editorial in the *Journal of Nursing Scholarship*, as pertinent then as it is today, Meleis wrote that there are multiple ways to define empowerment. One example she shares is what the United States and other developed countries are doing when they recruit nurses from less developed countries to work as nurses. It is a form of empowerment for these nurses to have the choice of where they would like to work. Meleis' perspective of empowerment involves giving nurses opportunities to use high technology, work in best-practice environments, increase their earning power, expand their education and knowledge base, and improve their families' overall situations. Certainly, through foreign recruitment, nurses are able to enjoy improved working conditions and improve their economic earning power. This perspective can be a win-win situation for all by empowering foreign nurses and their families, as well as the health care system in the developed country.

STRATEGIES TO EMPOWER ONESELF AND OTHERS

Another way to view empowerment is as "an interpersonal process of providing the resources, tools, and environment to develop, build, and increase ability and effectiveness of others to set and reach goals for individual and social ends" (Hokanson-Hawks, 1992, p. 610). A significant point is that nurses who do not have the resources to perform their jobs, no matter how good their self-esteem is and how aware they are of their poor situations, will not be able to complete their work. This aspect of empowerment, however, is generally assumed—that is, that nurses will have the basic resources to perform their work. Also significant for nurse empowerment is the idea that employers are often challenged to motivate their employees. So how do managers increase employee motivation, work performance, and effectiveness? Is there a best method? How does one motivate someone else? These are tough questions that have always concerned and challenged managers.

Jon Katzenbach (2003) writes extensively on employee motivation and how to best tap unused employee capabilities by empowering them. Energizing people to do their best work so as to accomplish higher goals than anyone thought possible is what happens when the group is empowered. Katzenbach presents five paths for energizing a workforce to generate high performance. He advocates that, before choosing one of the five paths, leaders need to conduct three reviews:

1. Review each of the five paths that can lead to having an emotionally committed, high-performing workforce. Identify what each has in common. Describe their differences. Brainstorm what conditions would favor following one path over another.
2. Determine why so many top-performing companies and institutions (the author presents in his book findings from studying several companies such as Southwest Airlines, Marriott, and Microsoft) follow different paths. Describe how the company was successful.
3. Determine how companies decide which path to follow.

These are Katzenbach's five paths:

- *Mission, values, and pride.* This path is favored by companies that have successful teams with a history of employee pride. There must be value-driven leadership. Some groups that align with this path are the U.S. Marine Corps and Marriott International.
- *Process and metrics.* This path best serves companies with maturing marketplace conditions that pride themselves for continuously improving. They are driven by a dynamic market and large customer base. Examples of groups using this path are Avon Manufacturing, Hill's Pet Nutrition, and Johnson Controls.
- *Entrepreneurial spirit.* These groups thrive on high-risk, high-reward opportunities. There are significant employee ownership possibilities. The groups are rapidly growing and enjoy a dynamic market. Most have magnetic leaders with ambitious visions for the companies. An example is Vail Ski School.
- *Individual achievement.* There are highly ambitious individuals employed in these groups, and individual achievement is of primary importance to the group. They tend to have an extremely dynamic marketplace and a huge customer base. Home Depot and First USA are examples of companies choosing this path.
- *Recognition and celebration.* It is critical that the average worker contributes. The labor pool tends to be unskilled with low monetary reward. The work itself tends not to be stimulating; however, there are magnetic leaders who trigger the energy of the workforce. Examples are Kentucky Fried Chicken and Southwest Airlines.

Katzenbach recommends that no matter what path is chosen, those in administration have to demonstrate that "they really care about each worker, and they have to honestly believe that he or she matters to the performance of the enterprise" (p. 236). He also notes that, although each organization that he studied focused predominantly on one path, they tended to use other paths as supplements to accomplishing work goals. It is imperative to realize that, in order to empower employees to be top performers, the leader-administrator must know how to generate emotional energy, how to channel the energy to be effective, and instill the discipline needed to maintain energy and commitment at such extraordinary levels. This model for motivating employees is very conducive for mentoring.

On the front cover of his book, *Why Pride Matters More Than Money*, Katzenbach (2003) dangles the infamous carrot. He believes emotional commitment from employees is the key to success and keeping competitive. Pride in one's work and recognition are significant rewards that nurses are seeking today. Many think that monetary reward is what it takes to motivate employees, but this is only part of it. Katzenbach (2003) repeatedly talks about pride. He feels that, in order to be successful and perform at a high level, one needs a strong ego as well as self-serving pride. Nursing, in any specialty area, is a high-performance job. If nurses can (1) feel proud of themselves and (2) have those they respect and admire feel proud of them, two motivational dimensions are satisfied. Katzenbach challenges all "leaders in almost any organizational setting to motivate higher employee performance by capitalizing on the anticipation of feeling proud and making others proud, too" (p. 3). He believes that development of pride-building skills can be learned and can build long-term sustainability for an organization. In addition, cultivating pride in the nursing workforce can propel the nursing profession to bigger and better things.

Risher (2003) lists four "common sense" ways of improving employee performance: (1) get the employees to work harder; (2) train them with better work methods to be more productive; (3) try to reengineer the way the work is done, and then train them again; and (4) empower the workers to develop better methods. Empowering employees involves trust, and once there is trust between the management and the employees, there will be increased performance. This is a new empowerment philosophy that recognizes what employees have to offer more so than ever before. Also, the idea of Total Quality Management, introduced by Deming (1994), assisted in demonstrating that frontline workers play a major role in solving quality problems. Along with this paradigm— trusting the worker—came a new focus on employee commitment, which Becker, Ulrich, and Houselid (2001) describe as "engagement plus dedication;" meaning that employees who are committed to the goals of the organization and have pride in their work will be intentionally engaged and willing to put in discretionary energy to accomplish their work goals. It is important to have employees who are committed to the organization and the profession, and not just to their own careers. Nurses, both mentors and mentees, can role model empowering behavior by

- being positive and proactive
- giving control to frontline employees
- offering culturally sensitive assistance
- encouraging individuals and recognizing all of the person's existing strengths
- increasing awareness of available support systems
- attempting to convey a joint sense of responsibility for work so a person does not become stressed
- promoting the use of coping strategies to prevent a sense of panic
- helping the person not only see that problems have been solved or needs met but that the person functioned as an active, responsible agent who played a significant role (Dunst & Trivette, 1987)

Books such as *201 Careers in Nursing* (Fitzpatrick & Ea, 2012) are resources to assist nurses and student nurses to make changes in their life through empowerment. Sullivan (2004) writes that becoming influential can be learned. In her book, *How to Be Influential as a Nurse*, she discusses strategies and techniques to assist nurses in enhancing their skills so they can become more influential wherever they work and in whatever position they hold. Becoming more influential is empowering. Hudacek's *A Daybook for Nurses: Making a Difference Each Day* (2004) explains how nurses have been empowered by their patients or their patients' families to make a difference that not only assisted one patient but made a difference for many patients. An excellent example that clearly depicts someone making a difference is a nurse who put an unstable premature twin in the newborn nursery bassinet with her stable, healthier twin to comfort and support her. The outcome was positive, and today this practice is universally implemented in neonatal intensive care units throughout the country.

Other resources also come into play here. Houser and Player (2004) recount the careers of 12 nurses (including Luther Christman, Gretta Styles, Loretta Ford, and Sue Donaldson) who became leaders in the profession. T. Miller (2003) presents ideas on developing a résumé to best portray one's expertise, skill set, and experiences. A. Miller (2002) also feels that just writing down one's abilities assists in improving one's self-confidence. In this light, he suggests that nurses practice their interviewing skills with each other or an adviser prior to seeking a position. For students, Miller advocates mentoring in three areas:

- Developmental (self-esteem, social skills, motivation, attitude, and behavioral changes)
- Work related (individual goals, work skills) and subject (lifelong learning philosophy, career)
- General academic goals

Certainly, assessing the work culture of organizations that new graduates are interested in working for is important, as Sirgo and Coeling (2005) note. They point to the importance of evaluating organizational culture and describe this as "how things are done around here." They suggest using their tool as a framework in evaluating the health of the work environment.

There are innovative ways to manage a career, such as having multiple career paths instead of just one job, working per diem to gain skills in a new clinical area, getting involved with health teaching outside the health care structure, such as teaching first aid at a marina, offering cardiopulmonary resuscitation certification for police or interested civilians, managing a website that answers new mothers' questions on infant care, writing a column in a newspaper or magazine, participating in research trial evaluations, or learning sales techniques to market pharmaceuticals or high-technology equipment.

Gilley and Boughton (1996) describe how the manager yields control to the staff and how this empowers both staff and the manager. "Self-esteeming" is a two-way process between two individuals. Increased self-confidence occurs after receiving positive evaluations from one's supervisor or colleagues. This, in turn, increases one's self-esteem. This self-esteeming for the employee takes the relationship to a much deeper level: "In return for receiving some control, the employee must now challenge and stimulate the manager with regard to his or her role and responsibility, which will create a higher level of confidence for the manager" (pp. 85–86). This is termed *reciprocal self-esteem*. It is an example of how nurses and managers can be synergistic and accomplish more at the same time that they improve staff morale. These authors offer a tool for measuring nurses' self-esteem as well as a checklist to determine outcomes of mentor-mentee relationships.

It is significant that the mentor or leader/manager also is empowered through the self-esteeming process. This process does not work if the nurse manager or mentor thinks, "I am only a nurse," or, "my nurses need to follow the doctor's orders period," or, "there is no need to call and ask about that patient; just follow the protocol that Dr. Lisa gave us." In fact, someone who is not empowered has no possibility of empowering, let alone assisting others to empower themselves. Shaffer, Tallarico, and Walsh (2000, p. 36) remind us that mentoring can assist colleagues who may feel "powerless and insignificant" in their health care system to gain pride and self-confidence from their mentoring and from the mentee. If there is a network of multiple mentors, along with peer mentoring, the culture of mentoring can become pervasive. Mentors gain leadership and teaching skills and rekindle their pride in the profession through a novice's eyes. Also, institutions are more likely to retain nurses who are feeling valued and empowered. However, Zachary (2009) feels that a mentor must want to be a mentor in order to be successful and feel they are part of the empowerment process of new employees and peers. It stands to reason that individuals who are not willing to mentor or who are manipulative will work against developing a mentoring culture in a unit.

Yeomans (1998) echoes what we all know to be true: the more one orders a person to do something a certain way, the better the chance is that it will be done in a less acceptable way. It is obvious that by using a participatory, not an autocratic, leadership style, one will best create an environment conducive to empowering staff. As Blanchard and Johnson (1982) describe in their classic work, *The One Minute Manager*, people who feel good about who they are produce the best results. Worrell, McGinn, Black, Holloway, and Ney (1996) propose the following model for faculty to role-model in order to provide empowerment to students, who will thereby become collegial, effective communicators, autonomous, and accountable:

- *Collegiality.* The relationship should be based on mutual respect for all involved. Faculty need to give honest feedback to students and not offer false praise in order to please them. Faculty should coach the students in order to use all of their potential. This acts to empower them. Faculty can also mentor their students by teaching them political survival skills.
- *Communication.* Faculty should effectively transmit information to all involved. There must be opportunities for students to engage in dialogue with their professors. Faculty cannot just provide all of the information that students need to learn. There must be interactive learning. Students who are spoon-fed information will be enabled and will not develop self-confidence.
- *Autonomy.* Students need to be independent. They need to learn problem-solving skills so they can think critically and have supervised practice in providing solutions to problems they encounter. Having autonomy will also increase student self-esteem.

- *Accountability.* Students must be responsible for their actions as well as their learning. Faculty or supervisors must not allow students to be rescued. They need to be held accountable for their actions. Faculty and supervisors who are codependent will offer unsolicited advice or enable a student who is actually capable of handling his or her own challenges. Table 3.1 presents some suggestions for individuals to use in order to increase their leadership skills and become or remain empowered.

The One Minute Manager by Blanchard and Johnson (1982) suggest some basic components of how to maximize an individual's empowerment that includes establishment of trust, genuine respect for one another, and an optimistic perspective about one's vision and goals. Success with this model revolves around developing an atmosphere of respect and recognition for the nurse that is totally transparent to all members of the health care team. DiMeglio et al. (2005) describe a mentor program they developed that concentrates on socializing new nurses. They discuss solutions regarding some of the issues that new nurses face, such as negative communication, generational differences, accountability, and peer competence. MacPhee et al. (2011) found in their study that if nurse leaders employ structural (having access to resources, good technological support, and communication networks) and psychological empowerment (intrinsic task motivation) processes there are higher nurse retention rates, increased commitment by nurses to the organization, and safer patient outcomes.

TABLE 3.1
Practice Strategies to Increase Staff Empowerment

Before registering a complaint, try to configure a possible solution that can be submitted along with the complaint

Stop whining about everything new. Be flexible, or at least try the change

Assess the pros and cons of the situation, and attempt to outweigh the cons

Prioritize one's battles. Focus on only the two most important ones

Review your colleagues' strengths

Review your own strengths

Avoid the doom and gloom. Try smiling, which releases endorphins and improves your overall well-being

Set a positive tone, and try to avoid peer pressure (when everyone agrees to something because someone else does and now are too tired to reflect comprehensively on the issue)

Network, and keep abreast of grassroot opinions

Empowerment is exactly what nurses need rather than being enabled to fulfill what the physician and others order for patients. The hierarchical structure that has existed for decades is changing, and staff nurses, advanced practice nurses, and nurse administrators are assuming more equitable positions of authority. Wheatley (2006) explains the new science of leadership and recommends empowering all and decreasing the constraints of bureaucratic structures. This organizational movement will generate higher-quality outcomes and improved patient care, therefore increasing productivity and decreasing costs, while improving the work environment. Among the benefits generated by nurse empowerment is improved patient care, increased nurse professionalism, and expanded nurse problem-solving ability (Espeland & Shanta, 2001).

ENABLING

Enabling is a perpetuation of the status quo and maintaining nurse dependency. Behavior that prevents an individual from acquiring new competencies, decreases one's sense of control over life, and reinforces old, maladaptive behaviors such as passivity and procrastination reflect enabling (Dunst & Trivette, 1987). In fact, enabling is defined by the field of drug and alcohol addiction as allowing or encouraging the drug dependence to continue or even worsen. Essentially, enabling is part of codependency. Someone who is codependent manifests behaviors of assuming others' responsibilities, taking care of others' needs, and rescuing others from the consequences of their behaviors. Faculty, managers, and colleagues can be guilty of protecting and rescuing certain students and nurses. Enabling is clearly described as a negative process used by individuals to reinforce an other person's dependency.

Enabling leads to people feeling entitled; that is, believing they should receive an honor or recognition because of the work they put into a project, or in preparing for a specific role in a play, or in practicing for selection to an elite athletic competition. One may hear nurses say, "I have paid my dues and refuse to work another Christmas holiday; let the new people do the holidays." This is a projection of feeling entitled and may be a result of having been enabled. An example of enabling follows.

Tom is a new BSN graduate who started his first RN position on a high acuity medical infectious disease unit, and keeps complaining about his BSN program. He complains that he never had exposure to any infectious disease patients except individuals with AIDS who were hospitalized for problems other than their AIDS status. He continuously told his preceptor he had never worked with patients with Lyme disease, meningitis, encephalitis, or even methicillin-resistant *Staphylococcus aureus* (MRSA) or vancomycin-resistant enterococci (VRE) infected patients. When called upon by his unit manager as to why he was not familiar with MRSA or VRE infections, his comments were: "I did not take care of the patients' infections, my instructor had me focus on their diabetes or cardiac disease." He also said that he was never taught in class about either of these commonly seen infectious states. When asked why he had not researched the infectious states on his own he commented: "I was supposed to have this information in school and I was not prepared adequately—this is extra work that I would have to do at home and I have too many other responsibilities. Plus, why should I research them at home and not get any payment for my time? I don't understand why my preceptor doesn't teach me what I need to know to do the job."

As one can easily see, Tom likes to blame his ignorance on everyone but himself and does not have the motivation to take responsibility for gaining the knowledge and experience he needs to acquire to fulfill his RN position. He was probably enabled all through his BSN program and has developed a habit to blame his ignorance on others and always have an excuse for not being prepared. He needs to be empowered to want to learn for learning's sake and become passionate about his role and becoming an effective RN.

Leaders need to empower students and nurses by teaching them to handle their own responsibilities, assisting them to become independent, and maintaining the policies of the hospital or health care agency or school of nursing so they have to face the consequences of their actions. Faculty must provide opportunities for students to do their own problem solving and be accountable for them; otherwise, student self-esteem will suffer, and they will never become empowered.

RECOGNITION AND PRIDE GENERATED FROM HEALTHY WORK ENVIRONMENTS

Kouzes and Posner (2003) suggest that people who are recognized for their good work and are encouraged are more likely to achieve higher levels of success. They recommend strategies for leaders to use to support others' needs to be appreciated for what they do. They explain "encouraging the heart" as consisting of four components:

- Leaders must follow general principles that reward employees for work well done
- Leaders will not be perceived as being soft for encouraging the heart. In fact, in order to fulfill stretch goals, it is essential to follow the heart
- Various leaders have multiple methods they use to encourage the heart
- All leaders must be aware of the soul and spirit involved in any organization

Just as Sinetar (1998) describes mentoring as the art of encouragement and soul, Kouzes and Posner (2003) note that an extremely important component of empowering staff is to "encourage the heart," such as the encouragement a mentor gives. This encouragement of the heart is often what is missing in the work environment of nurses, yet is a spirit that fits with advancing a mentoring culture in nursing.

The American Association of Critical-Care Nurses (AACN) (2005) developed six evidence-based standards that constitute a healthy work environment. These include: skilled communication, true collaboration, effective decision making, adequate staffing, meaningful recognition, and authentic leadership, and are correlated with high RN retention and staff job satisfaction. The AACN also developed a tool to use to measure healthy work environments that can be accessed off the AACN website, www.hweteamtool.org/main/index (AACN, 2010). Vollers, Hill, Roberts, Dambaugh, and Brenner (2009) describe how the *AACN Healthy Work Environment Policy* fosters successful empowerment of RNs and the entire staff. Helton (2009) shares an example of her ICU unit that adapted the AACN's Health Work Environment Model and created a mentoring program, critical care internship, Stars of the Month Recognition of Staff Nurses Program, and clinical newsletter that all served to increase staff empowerment.

Receiving recognition has consistently been an identified factor that nurses perceive as highly correlated to high job satisfaction. Some methods of recognition of staff nurses include the opportunity to serve on a task force, receiving additional training to share with peers, preceptorships, participation in unit orientation, involvement in planning for patient care or the unit operation, having charge nurse responsibilities, or an invitation to speak at a professional meeting.

Cohen, Stuenkel, and Nguyen (2009) used the *Revised Nursing Work Index* (NWI–R) and also found that staff retention and job satisfaction of staff nurses are highly correlated with a healthy work environment. The NWI-R measures professional autonomy, collaborative relationships with physicians and nurses, access to resources, leadership ability of managers, and organizational support (Lake & Frieese, 2006). Additionally, job satisfaction and increased RN retention are improved when these nurses perceive their nurse managers manifest strong leadership characteristics (Duffield, Roche, Blay, & Stase, 2011). Mentors and preceptors can assist their colleagues in gaining leadership skills by giving them opportunities to practice effective communication, administrative tasks, team building, conflict management, and supervision of other employees—for example, by

- taking positions that offer new and increased responsibilities
- managing special start-up assignments that afford them visibility
- handling personnel problems like conflicts and firings
- representing the unit at a division or departmental meeting
- leading a unit staff meeting
- scheduling and managing staff work requests for the next 3-month period
- developing an interdisciplinary clinical protocol
- meeting with members of outside health care agencies to set up a partnership

Bernhard and Walsh (1990) provide an interesting four-stage model that integrates and substantiates the close relationship between mentoring, empowering, and motivating individuals:

- *Stage 1, Input.* Employees must have inner motivation in order for mentoring and empowerment to occur.
- *Stage 2, Process.* Through mentoring, energy can be channeled to accomplish goals and increase mentees' perceptions of the environment. Both the mentor and mentee become motivated to achieve their own goals.
- *Stage 3, Output.* The goal of mentoring is for the mentee to become empowered. This prepares the mentee to be accountable.
- *Stage 4, Feedback.* The empowered mentee will acquire high self-esteem and competence. It is time for the mentee to mentor and attempt to motivate someone else.

This model could be helpful for managers to use when illustrating the process a mentor and mentee can expect with the progression of a mentoring relationship. It also spells out the cyclical nature of mentoring on a unit or department. The stages of input, process, output, and feedback can be put on a horizontal continuum and dated so that the mentor and mentee have target dates for their completion of the mentorship.

It is imperative that nurses be empowered to become leaders, and mentoring can strengthen this initiative. Currently, each individual nurse is expected to be a leader and to have some degree of some type(s) of power. Power can be shared to help others and specific individuals have more or less power depending on the situation. This is the essence of empowerment. In order to empower nurses on a unit, a nurse manager has to provide mentoring relationships and give nurses freedom to use their creativity to generate new ideas and accomplish goals. Nurses can empower each other and share their power through mentoring and networking with each other. Aiken et al. (2010) document that nurses need to be more collaborative with peers and other members of the health care team, more autonomous with their decision making, and more capable of providing strong leadership. How better to learn collaboration skills, gain self-confidence, increase decision-making ability, and develop leadership than to work with a coach or mentor?

Shaffer et al. (2000) suggest the following actions be included in order for successful empowerment of mentor and mentee during the traditional stages of the mentoring relationship:

1. *Initiation.* During this initial time, the two people should determine the other's qualities that interest each in forming the mentorship. For example, what strengths and networks does the mentor have? What potential does the mentor see in the mentee? What is in it for the mentor? Ideas for establishing goals are discussed.
2. *Cultivation.* The relationship is defined with specific goals and activities that will benefit both mentor and mentee. Are there any connections that the mentor or mentee may have to expedite the accomplishments of goals? Schedules are made that are mutually agreed on by both the mentor and mentee.
3. *Separation.* Some mentorships end spontaneously, but most that are successful enter this phase, and both the mentor and the mentee gradually dissolve or limit the relationship. Often one of the two experiences a career move that separates them geographically, but they remain in a long-term relationship in spite of the distance. They continue to assist each other with career advancement and are now more like colleagues, both being equally empowered.
4. *Redefinition.* This stage varies with each pair, and some relationships never proceed to this stage because they just end. It is

difficult to know if the mentee or mentor were ever empowered if the mentoring relationship did not progress and faded away. Others become colleagues and enjoy success from their relationship. There is little advice being given at this point since the pair have most likely become peers who are equally empowered and are both richer for their mentorship.

One mentoring program for senior nurse executives, the Executive Nurse Fellows Program, for the Robert Wood Johnson Foundation, developed by the Center for the Health Professions at the University of California, San Francisco, has been experimenting with the most effective ways nurses can change their skill sets in order to more fully participate in delivering health care. Nurses need to be prepared to assist with the reintegration of psychosocial behavioral aspects of care with the traditional biomedical ones, the design of creative teams to participate effectively in care delivery systems, and the redesign of care delivery systems to maximize patient outcomes.

The Leadership Program described by O'Neil and Morjikian (2003) encompasses five competencies that each executive (and nurses wishing to increase their leadership skills) must master during the fellowship:

- *Self-knowledge*, defined as the ability to develop the self in the context of organizational challenges and interpersonal demands.
- *Interpersonal communication effectiveness*, which encompasses the ability to translate a vision and motivate followers. Followers engage in exercises to assist them in understanding how they are perceived by others.
- *Risk taking and creativity*, so as to move beyond what has worked in the past and develop transformational changes to move the organization to success.
- *Inspiring change* in order to steer the organization in an entirely different way that provides maximum effectiveness.
- *Strategic vision for the future*, so that connections between social, economic, and political issues are a part of the organization's long-term plan.

Participants use self-ratings and peer and supervisor ratings to gather data and to map out a development plan for their year as a fellow. Coaches as well as other fellows and peers assist each other in determining their plan of leadership development. Lombardo and Eichinger (2004) give some specific strategies for the fellow as well as the coaches and mentors in their book, *For Your Improvement: A Development and*

Coaching Guide. Although this is designed as an advanced leadership program for nurse executives in health services, public health, and nursing education, anyone can gain leadership skills by practicing these strategies, and mentors can role model them for mentees. Sandler (2011) also offers some helpful strategies for executives using the psychodynamic approach, with the aim to have the executives improve their performance at work for their organizations and for their own professional gains. Specific ideas for assisting nurses to achieve excellence are described by Campbell, Gilbert, and Lausten (2010).

What nurse executives and managers may feel they are exemplifying as their leadership style is not always perceived similarly by staff. This is a good reason to participate in a leadership development seminar in order to attain feedback on how one's communication and leadership styles are perceived by others. Certainly among the biggest challenges nurses face are communication and collaboration problems. For example, a tool to measure nurse–physician communication found that nurses working in a unit that had high patient safety concerns had the least effective physician–nurse communication as perceived by the nurses (Manojlovich et al., 2011). Thomas, Sexton, and Helmreich (2003) found a difference between nurse and physician perceptions of communication among health care members. They found that 73% of the physicians felt there was a high quality of collaboration with nurses, but only 33% of the nurses agreed that they a had high-quality collaboration with physicians. Rosenstein (2002) found with 1,200 responses from employees of 84 hospitals and medical groups in the Veterans Hospital Agency West Coast network that there was a discrepancy between nurses and physicians regarding the professional atmosphere at their facilities. There was a statistically significant difference, with physicians feeling they enjoyed good collaboration and nurses feeling they did not. In fact, 30% of respondents felt they knew at least one nurse who had left the institution because of disruptive, noncollegial physician behavior.

The American Colleges of Collegiate Nursing sponsors a year-long leadership fellowship for nurse faculty interested in becoming deans and directors of nursing programs. Approximately 50 fellows are selected annually and attend two 3-day workshops in Washington, D.C., where they participate in leadership development groups and work with a dean mentor throughout the year (for information on the fellowship and application process, go to www.aacn.nche.edu). This fellowship affords the opportunity for leadership assessment and evaluation, networking, and consultation with a mentor to achieve long-term goals.

International mentoring through the Chiron Mentor-Fellow Program was another mentoring program that has advanced nursing as well as individual nurse's careers. Sigma Theta Tau International (STTI) offers members the opportunity to work with mentors and develop leadership skills in a formalized fellowship through the Chiron Mentor-Fellow Program. During the 12-month program, nurses who desired skill development in specific leadership areas were guided by experienced mentors as they implemented individualized plans and participated in group activities.

Aiken et al. (2010) document that nurses need to be more collaborative with peers and other members of the health care team, more autonomous with their decision making, and more capable of providing strong leadership. Additionally, these researchers found that where there are mandatory staffing policies, such as in California, there is less patient mortality. Mentors can assist leaders to become empowered and be more collaborative, autonomous, and better leaders. Mentorships assist nurses in gaining insight into their ability to lead change, think creatively, empower themselves as well as others, and acquire skills to prepare them for a successful career and strengthen the nursing profession. Nurses identify that it is most significant for the nurse manager and other leaders to portray caring in order to have a healthy care environment that is conducive to staff empowerment (Burston & Stichler, 2010). Koloroutis (2004) agrees that caring is a significant attribute of an effective leader and describes how work settings can be more focused on caring in her book, *Relationship-Based Care: A Model for Transforming Practice*. Risher (2003) points out that the biggest problem for managers is to have employees who do not care about the success of the organization. This disengagement can be identified easily by looking for the people who put in their time and go home. Approximately one out of three employees feel this way. No one wants them as employees, but they can be found in every workplace (Risher, 2003). Another significant factor is the correlation of high job satisfaction of nurses and a collaborative team effort between staff (Kalisch, Lee, & Rochman, 2010). Increased job satisfaction of RNs was found when nurses perceived they were working within cohesive multidisciplinary teams (Kovner, Brewer, Wu, Cheng, & Suzuki, 2006).

Mentoring should be institutionalized as an integral part of nursing practice—as a useful, honorable way of life and a part of being a fully functional and professional nurse (Werner, 2002). Having a mentor can greatly assist every nurse to develop leadership ability. Nurses need to have good relationships among themselves in order to be a successful team. Team building must be focused on performance results and not just on creating a team. Katzenbach and Smith (2003) present basic rules for team building in their best seller, *The Wisdom of Teams: Creating the High-Performance Organization*:

- Have no more than 12 people on any team to ensure effectiveness
- The team must have a common purpose
- There must be a common set of specific performance goals
- There must be a commonly agreed on working approach
- All members must hold one another mutually accountable for their performance

The authors say that teams outperform individuals especially when performance requires multiple talents and types of experience. And although most people agree that teams almost always outperform individuals, they generally overlook opportunities to participate in teams, especially those in higher-level positions. The authors describe Jack Welch, former chief executive officer of General Electric, as saying everyone's job is to provide excellent customer service from the CEO to the receptionist.

Nurses need to get back to serving the customer. We all can benefit from working in teams, and Katzenbach and Smith (2003) explain why teams perform so well. First, working in a team brings together skills, experience, and knowledge that surpass what any one individual has. Second, a team can accomplish goals more quickly than any one individual. Third, teams are cost-effective. And finally, teams bring socialization into the work setting and tend to provide opportunities for fun, which solidifies teams further. Teams are related to networks, and as we know, networking triggers success in most people's work settings as well as careers. Coaches and mentors, such as clinical nurse specialists, staff development directors, and other department and special project directors, have a key role in assisting these teams to produce the maximum performance possible. One significant learning goal of people experiencing coaching sessions is to learn how to ask the most significant and powerful questions regarding one's career or issues confronting the organization that an individual is involved with (Stoltzfus, 2008).

Stone (1999), another well-known coach, offers some critical skills for team coaching:

- *Defining.* Direct the team to identify a purpose and goals.
- *Summarizing.* Summarize the team's progress at each milestone, and bring the team together to rework goals and evaluate work as necessary.

- *Facilitating.* Keep the team spirit alive by encouraging dialogue, but be sure not to assume leadership of the team. Stay in the facilitator role.
- *Organizing.* Distribute agendas, plan meetings, circulate minutes, and keep the team on track for accomplishing its goals.
- *Developing.* Role model the skills the team needs in order to work together to accomplish its goals.

How better to accomplish this than by role modeling for the new nurses, allowing nurses to shadow each other, providing a strong precepting program for skill orientation, and having a manager and staff who recognize each other's strengths and competencies? As Wheatley says, power is the result of the quality of the relationships that one has (2006). Nurses need to role-model more for each other the positive ways of communicating and managing conflict so that all nurses can be empowered to stand up and say what is really bothering them or what they would like to see happen where they work. This positive role modeling can generate an atmosphere in which nurses want to be mentored and choose to mentor. Growth will be encouraged and nurtured, and self-empowerment of nurses will be visible. This increased leadership ability of all nurses will increase patient care quality, cost-effectiveness, and nurse retention. As more and more networking generates collaboration between health care teams there will be more empowered individuals who will demonstrate higher performance.

Empowerment of a mentee is crucial to the success of a mentorship. However, the mentor must be self-empowered, as evidenced by exhibiting self-esteem and a positive self-image, being a risk taker and not dependent on the approval of others, having positive expectations, and being able to interact with others effectively (Lloyd & Berthelot, 2003). Many truly empowered and effective leaders say, "I have completed my job here when you no longer need me," which means the employees have become empowered.

CONCLUSION

Empowerment is necessary for all nurses as well as for the advancement of the profession of nursing. As leaders develop, they become more self-empowered and able to empower others. Nurses must gain self-confidence, a goal that can be achieved by becoming competent with both clinical skills and leadership skills such as negotiation, creative thinking, communication, and collaboration. In order to achieve this confidence, nurses need to be mentored by experienced nurses who can provide knowledge, psychosocial support, and networking. Mentors can assist individuals to increase their self-confidence, and in time, their self-esteem will heighten. By affording opportunities for nurses to empower themselves, practice leadership, and work with role models, coaches, and mentors, nurses will continue to make a difference in patient care.

REFERENCES

Aiken, L. H., Sloane, D. M., Cimiotti, J. P., Clarke, S., Flynn, L., Seago, J. A., ... Smith, H. L. (2010). Implications of the California nurse staffing mandate for other states. *Health Service Research, 45*(4), 904–921.

American Association of Critical-Care Nurses. (2005). *AACN standards for establishing and sustaining health work environments.* Retrieved from http://www.aacn.org/WD/HWE/Docs/HWEStandards.pdf

American Association of Critical-Care Nurses. (2010). *Tool to measure healthy work environments.* Retrieved from www.hweteamtool.org/main/index

Becker, B., Ulrich, D., & Houselid, M. (2001). *The human resource scorecard: Linking people, strategy, and performance.* Boston, MA: Harvard Business School Press.

Bernhard, L., & Walsh, M. (1990). *Leadership: The key to the professionalization of nursing* (2nd ed.). St. Louis, MO: Mosby.

Blanchard, K., & Johnson, S. (1982). *The one minute manager.* New York, NY: Berkeley.

Bradshaw, A. (1995). What are nurses doing to patients? A review of theories of nursing past and present. *Journal of Clinical Nursing, 4,* 81–92.

Burston, P. L., & Stichler, J. F. (2010). Nursing work environment and nurse caring: Relationship among motivational factors. *Journal of Advanced Nursing, 66*(8), 1819–1831.

Campbell, M., Gilbert, M., & Lausten, G. (2010). *Clinical coaching for nursing excellence.* Philadelphia, PA: F. A. Davis.

Cohen, J., Stuenkel, D., & Nguyen, Q. (2009). Providing a healthy work environment for nurses: The implications on retention. *Journal of Nursing Care Quarterly, 24,* 308–315.

Deming, W. E. (1994). *The new economics for industry, government, and education* (2nd ed.). Cambridge, MA: MIT Center for Advanced Engineering.

DiMeglio, K., Padula, C., Piatek, C., Korber, S., Barrett, A., Ducharme, M., ... Corry, K. (2005). Group cohesion and nurse satisfaction: Examination of a team-building approach. *Journal of Nursing Administration, 35,* 110–120.

Duffield, C. M., Roche, M. A., Blay, N. & Stase, H. (2011). Nursing unit managers, staff retention and the work environment. *Journal of Clinical Nursing, 20*(1–2), 23–25.

Dunst, C., & Trivette, C. (1987). Enabling and empowering families: Conceptual and intervention issues. *School Psychology Review, 16,* 443–456.

Espeland, K. & Shanta, L. (2001). Empowering versus enabling in academia. *Journal of Nursing Education, 40,* 342–346.

Fitzpatrick, J., & Ea, E. (2012). *201 careers in nursing.* New York, NY: Springer.

Gershon, D., & Straub, G. (2011). *Empowerment: The art of creating your life as you want it.* Hurley, NY: Highpoint.

Gilley, J., & Boughton, N. (1996). *Stop managing, start coaching.* Chicago, IL: Irwin.

Grossman, S., & Valiga, T. (2009). *The new leadership challenge: Creating the future of nursing* (3rd ed.). Philadelphia, PA: F. A. Davis.

Helton, R. E. (2009). In our unit: Creating a healthy work environment. *Critical Care Nurse, 29*(5), 80, 78–79.

Hokanson-Hawks, J. (1992). Empowerment in nursing education: Concept analysis and application to philosophy, learning and instruction. *Journal of Advanced Nursing, 17,* 609–618.

Houser, B., & Player, K. (2004). *Pivotal moments in nursing: Leaders who changed the path of a profession.* Indianapolis, IN: STTI.

Hudacek, S. (2004). *A daybook for nurses: Making a difference each day.* Indianapolis, IN: Center Nursing Press.

Kalisch, B. J., Lee, H., & Rochman, M. (2010). Nursing staff teamwork and job satisfaction. *Journal of Nursing Management, 18,* 938–947.

Katzenbach, J. (2003). *Why pride matters more than money: The power of the world's greatest motivational force.* New York, NY: Crown Business.

Katzenbach, J., & Khan, Z. (2010). *Leading outside the lines: How to mobilize the (in)formal organization, energize your team and get better results.* San Francisco, CA: Jossey-Bass.

Katzenbach, J., & Smith, D. (2003). *The wisdom of teams: Creating the high performance organization* (2nd ed.). New York, NY: HarperCollins.

Kodish, E., Eder, M., Noll, R., Ruccione, K., Lange, B., Angiolillo, A., ... Drotar, D. (2004). Communication of randomization in childhood leukemia trials. *Journal of the American Medical Association, 291,* 470–475.

Koloroutis, K. (Ed.). (2004). *Relationship-based care: A model for transforming practice.* Minneapolis, MN: Creative Health Care Management.

Kouzes, J., & Posner, B. (2003). *Encouraging the heart: A leader's guide to rewarding and recognizing others* (2nd ed.). San Francisco, CA: Jossey-Bass.

Kouzes, J., & Posner, B. (2007). *The leadership challenge* (4th ed.). San Francisco, CA: Jossey-Bass.

Kovner, C., Brewer, C., Wu, Y. W., Cheng, Y., & Suzuki, M. (2006). Factors associated with work satisfaction of registered nurses. *Journal of Nursing Scholarship, 38,* 71–79.

Lake, E. T., & Frieese, C. R. (2006). Variations in nursing practice environments: Relation to staffing and hospital characteristics. *Nursing Research, 55,* 1–9.

Lloyd, S. R., & Berthelot, T. (2003). *Self empowerment* (2nd ed.). Los Altos, CA: Crisp Publications.

Lombardo, M., & Eichinger, R. (2004). *For your improvement: A development and coaching guide* (4th ed.). Minneapolis, MN: Lominger.

MacPhee, M., Skelton-Green, J., Bouthillette, F., & Suryaprakash, N. (2011). An empowerment framework for nursing leadership development: Supporting evidence. *Journal of Advanced Nursing, 68*(1), 159–169.

Manojlovich, M., Saint, S., Forman, J., Fletcher, C., Keith, R., & Krein, S. (2011). Developing and testing a tool to measure nurse/physician communication in the intensive care unit. *Journal of Patient Safety, 7*(2), 80–84.

Meleis, A. (2003). Brain drain or empowerment? *Journal of Nursing Scholarship, 35,* 105.

Miller, A. (2002). *Mentoring students and young people.* Sterling, VA: Stylus Publishing.

Miller, T. (2003). *Building and managing a career in nursing: Strategies for advancing your career.* Indianapolis, IN: STTI.

O'Neil, E., & Morjikian, R. (2003). Nursing leadership: Challenges and opportunities. *Policy, Politics, and Nursing Practice, 4,* 173–179.

Risher, H. (2003). Tapping unused employee capabilities: How to create a high performance environment by changing the work paradigm. *Public Manager, 32,* 34–39.

Roberts, D., & Vasquez, E. (2004). Power: An application to the nursing image and advanced practice. *AACN Clinical Issues, 15,* 196–204.

Rosenstein, A. (2002). Original research: Nurse-physician relationships: Impact on nurse satisfaction and retention. *American Journal of Nursing, 102,* 26–34.

Sandler, C. (2011). *Executive coaching: A psychodynamic approach.* Berkshire, England: McGraw-Hill.

Shaffer, B., Tallarico, B., & Walsh, J. (2000). Win-win mentoring. *Dimensions of Critical Care Nursing, 6,* 36–38.

Sinetar, M. (1998). *The mentor's spirit: Life lessons on leadership and the art of encouragement.* New York, NY: St. Martin's Press.

Sirgo, C., & Coeling, H. (2005). Work group culture and the new graduate. *American Journal of Nursing, 105,* 85–87.

Starhawk. (2011). *The empowerment manual: A guide for collaborative groups.* Gabriola Island, BC: New Society Publishers.

Stoltzfus, T. (2008). *Coaching questions: A coach's guide to powerful asking skills.* Virginia Beach, VA: T. Stoltzzfus.

Stone, F. (1999). *Coaching, counseling, and mentoring: How to choose and use the right technique to boost employee performance.* New York, NY: AMACON.

Sullivan, E. (2004). *How to be influential as a nurse.* Upper Saddle River, NJ: Prentice Hall.

Thomas, E., Sexton, B., & Helmreich, R. (2003). Discrepant attitudes about teamwork among critical care nurses and physicians. *Critical Care Medicine, 31,* 956–959.

Vollers, D., Hill, E., Roberts, C., Dambaugh, L., & Brenner, Z. R. (2009). AACN's healthy work environment standards and an empowering nurse advancement system. *Critical Care Nurse, 29*(6), 20–27.

Werner, J. (2002). Mentoring and its potential nursing role. *Creative Nursing Journal, 3,* 13–14.

Wheatley, M. (2006). *Leadership and the new science: Discovering order in a chaotic world* (3rd ed.). San Francisco, CA: Berrett-Koehler.

Worrell, J., McGinn, A., Black, E., Holloway, N., & Ney, P. (1996). The RN-BSN student: Developing a model of empowerment. *Journal of Nursing Education, 35*, 127–130.

Yeomans, W. (1998). *7 survival skills for a re-engineered world*. New York, NY: Penguin Publishing.

Zachary, L. (2009). *The mentee's guide: Making mentoring work for you*. San Francisco, CA: Jossey-Bass.

4

Strategies for Developing Mentorships in Nursing: One Size Does Not Fit All

Mentoring, a crucial skill and service to the profession, should be promoted among professional nurses, considered a leadership competency in clinical practice for all nurses, and integrated into the nursing curriculum. It is important for individual nurses to identify skills they wish to work on and then choose someone to work with who possesses those attributes or skills. In brief, we must we must mentor nurses in order to create leaders. Other related leadership skills— managing conflict, maintaining credibility, communicating effectively, taking risks, being flexible, being creative, having visions, and critically thinking—are important for leaders to assist individuals to develop. Given the state of flux in the health care industry, nurses are constantly considering new and more cost-effective ways of providing care. Collaborating, partnering, and networking skills are vital to ensuring the success of such developing health care delivery methods.

It is helpful at this point, however, to review the idea of a learning organization, which promotes continuous dialogue among its constituents. Senge, Kleiner, Roberts, Ross, and Smith remind us in their classic book, *The Fifth Discipline Fieldbook: Strategies and Tools for Building a Learning Organization,* that "a person is a person because of other people's acknowledgement" (1994, p. 3). Individuals who grow up with this idea—that we need others to successfully form our identities—are aware of the need for creating a mentoring culture. Five recommended learning disciplines follow for individuals to use when fostering this team effort attitude (from Senge et al.):

1. *Personal mastery.* Encouraging members of organizational settings to develop themselves around their individual goals and purposes.

2. *Mental models.* Attempting to continually clarify our internal pictures of the world that influences our actions and decisions.
3. *Shared vision.* Being part of a group by building a sense of commitment toward shared futures.
4. *Team learning.* Honing thinking skills so that groups of people "can reliably develop intelligence and ability greater than the sum of individual members' talents" (p. 6).
5. *Systems thinking.* A way of rethinking about how forces and interrelationships shape the behavior of systems to be more synchronized with the larger processes of the world.

Developing mentorships, coaching relationships, and preceptorships that reflect these five disciplines can be helpful in improving nurse morale and help to solidify the profession's contributions to health care. Leaders can make a difference by asking other nurses to follow a lifelong learning philosophy by modeling the behaviors in the five disciplines. Senge, Scharmer, Jaworski, and Flowers (2004) also share their ideas on collaboration and networking in order to create a preferred future. Nurses need direction in finding ways to create change and ultimately the future. One important belief is to acknowledge that nurses must work with others to be successful. Therefore, mentoring others through partnering initiatives will undoubtedly assist nurses to be more successful leaders and gain higher satisfaction with their professional and personal lives.

This chapter thus reviews characteristics for identifying successful mentors and mentees, how the generational gap impacts mentors and mentees, and effective mentoring, coaching, and precepting models. It also describes variables to assist with pairing of mentors and mentees. Since one size does not fit all, nurses need to be able to develop mentorships, preceptorships, and coaching styles to fit individuals and their work or personal situations. People vary according to their developmental stages, their levels of competency, their leadership and followership styles, and in other ways. Even with preceptorships with prescribed orientation programs and specific skill checklists, the preceptor needs to individualize the program to the preceptee.

CHARACTERISTICS OF EFFECTIVE MENTORS AND MENTEES

To be successful with mentorships of any kind, it stands to reason that the individuals who are going to be mentors or preceptors should be interested in mentoring or precepting others and possess certain characteristics. Tables 4.1 and 4.2, regarding mentoring within various models, are based on a review of the literature and will help in highlighting such characteristics (Allen, Eby, & Lentz, 2006; Andrews & Wallis, 1999; Bennetts, 2000; Byrne & Keefe, 2003; Greene & Puetzer, 2002; Schwiebert, 2000; White, 2007; Wilkes, 2006; Zachary, 2005, 2009).

It is important to note that there is agreement that mentors who fit this classification can still act negatively if they are manipulative and incompatible with their mentees. Indeed, some mentors may act as though everything is going along well with their mentoring but secretly abuse mentees to obtain more mileage for their own careers or even sabotage mentees' careers. A mentor may temporarily enable and protect a mentee who is not prepared sufficiently until enough time lapses that the mentor anticipates no further positive outcomes and ceases investing time and resources into the relationship. Some mentors, of course, view failure to mentor an individual successfully as their own failure and do not attribute it to the mentee or situation. Whether an ineffective mentoring or precepting relationship will be identified by others or the organization depends on several variables. With a preceptorship, when the time involved is limited and the goal is focused on attaining skills for orientation to a particular position, it can be difficult to evaluate if the precepting is good. However, if similar observations occur with this individual's preceptees, and they have not attained required skills, it is not too difficult to identify the preceptor as the problem. Another compounding variable is that preceptors generally have to precept new employees in order to maintain their clinical ladder positions or attain promotions on the clinical ladder. Having a mandate to precept can have a great impact on the relationship between the preceptor and preceptee since the preceptor, in many instances, has not voluntarily accepted this responsibility. To counteract possible deleterious aspects, or when ineffective precepting is obvious, it is advantageous if staff nurses can serve in another position, such as charge nurse, scheduler, or resource person.

As far as coaching goes, this is generally a short-term relationship that senior administrators assign to managers. The coach, who may be part of the organization or an outside consultant, nevertheless will be scrutinized by senior administration. The coach and coachee relationship is successful when the coachee's goals and senior administration's objectives are met.

Luna and Cullen (2000) believe that not every individual is a good mentee and not every individual needs a mentoring relationship. Others (Allen, Eby, Poteet, & Lentz, 2004; Bennetts, 2000; Schwiebert, 2000; Zachary, 2005, 2009) explain that everyone who has an effective mentor can benefit in some way(s) from the relationship. As previously discussed, most nurses have precepting relationships, not mentorships, and the precepting relationship has more of a skill-oriented focus over a defined period of time. Some preceptorships also focus on decision making and allow the preceptee to have continuous consultations with them even after the orientation period. Preceptees, of course, need to demonstrate satisfactory skills and decision-making abilities in their preceptorships in order to complete their orientations to becoming staff nurses. Due to the nature of a preceptorship, the preceptor and preceptee can generally work out any differences, whereas the relationship between a mentor and mentee is more intricate, and the behavior and productivity of mentees have a more direct reflection on the mentors. Coaches and those coached seem to be able to accomplish goals regarding the skills or knowledge that they are hoping to receive in their short-term relationships. It is most advantageous for the mentoring, precepting, or coaching relationship if both parties possess the characteristics listed in Tables 4.1 and 4.2.

TABLE 4.1
Characteristics of Effective Mentors

Strong self-esteem and self-empowerment

Effective communication skills

Uninvested in preserving the status quo

Politically astute in the workplace environment

Able to balance personal and professional responsibilities

Respected in the workplace by peers and senior administrators

Highly knowledgeable in the field and interested in new challenges

Willing to volunteer to mentor someone and past experience with a good mentor

effective mentoring experience

place considers mentoring significant and valuable

mentor well; there is incentive to be a good mentor, and resources the mentor

TABLE 4.2
Characteristics of Effective Mentees

Comfortable and willing to participate in mentorship

Effective communication skills

Willing to receive constructive feedback and work under the direction of another

Goal driven and with goals that are compatible with the mentor's goals

An area of interest that is different from but compatible with the mentor's expertise

Determination to succeed and passionate about the profession

Responsible and able to be an independent decision maker when appropriate

Flexible and willing to participate in low-level work initially that may directly assist the mentor or organization and not necessarily the mentee

THE GENERATIONAL IMPLICATIONS
FOR MENTORS AND MENTEES

The literature (Campbell & Campbell, 2009; Cary, 2008; Pitt-Catsouphes & Smyer, 2007; Sherman, 2006; Stewart, 2006) defines the various generations in this manner: (a) Traditionals (born between 1925–1945) possess a strong work ethic and are a product of the Great Depression; (b) Baby Boomers (born between 1946–1964) are highly competitive, willing to sacrifice now for success later, and are the product of living right after two world wars; (c) Generation Xers (1965–1980) value self-reliance, individualism, are loyal to themselves rather than the work setting, and are influenced by technology advances; (d) Millennials/Generation Y (1981–mid 90s) are very comfortable with technology, used to instant communication, have high expectations of self and workplace, and are drawn to their families for safety and security; and (e) Linksters (born after 1995) are the Facebook crowd, highly sophisticated and technologically skilled, tied to parents, very tolerant of alternative lifestyles, and involved in social activism. Given these differences, it is not hard to see why people from different generations working in the same setting can experience problems in communicating, expectations, and more.

In terms of specific differences between generations, Kupperschmidt (2006) points several out, except for the Linksters who are only 15 years (at the oldest) and so not involved in the work settings as of now: (a) The Traditionals follow orders and expect others to; (b) Baby

Boomers prefer to talk about how to get a task completed and are sure to get everyone to participate in the decision; (c) Generation X'ers want to do the task themselves at work; and (d) Generation Y'ers do no care so much as to who does the work as long as it is completed.

But how does this relate to mentoring? One will easily see that individuals within the various generations possess different strengths, so a multiple mentoring and/or peer mentoring model would be best for these individuals to maximize their talents and increase their abilities to respect each other and communicate more effectively. This would lead to a decrease in conflict and, hopefully, a more diverse and productive mentoring culture in work settings. Hurley and Snowden (2008) identify that the classic mentoring model may be effective, too, since the older and more experienced Traditionals and Baby Boomers have the knowledge and may require some empowerment to boost their self-confidence with working with the technologically savvy, although less experienced and knowledgeable Gen X'ers and Y'ers. These authors share how they used intergenerational mentoring to improve their organization. Others also stressed that intergenerational mentoring is a most effective way to assign mentors and mentees, either in preceptorships or coaching relationships or as peer mentors, as long as sufficient communication training has been conducted and all members of the unit/workforce are aware of intergenerational differences as well as how these differences can actually make the organization stronger (Brunetto, Farr-Wharton, & Shacklock, 2012). George, Whitehouse, and Whitehouse (2011) share their experiences working at a charter school and suggest that having this "intergenerativity" is a most favorable outcome of effective communication between members of the different generations and how powerful these intergenerational partnerships can be. Campbell and Campbell (2009) offer six strategies to use in the workplace to decrease conflict with employees of different generations involved, which can also be applied to mentor and mentees:

1. All should be aware of characteristics of different generations
2. Values and beliefs of each group should be clear
3. Members should share their perceptions
4. Consider pairing a Baby Boomer and Gen Y'er
5. Attempt to find some commonality between each member
6. Emphasize that both mentor and mentee can learn from each other

MENTORING MODELS

There are no standard mentoring models used in nursing that are universally accepted (Ensher & Murphy, 2005). Stages of mentoring have been described in Chapter 2 as including selection, goal setting, and working (Bower, 2000); recognition and development, limited independence, and termination and realignment (Fox & Shephard, 1998); and initiation, cultivation, separation, and redefinition (Kram, 1983). All seem to include similar components. Models in nursing do not correlate the stages of a mentoring relationship to any specific model. Rather, it is assumed that everyone proceeds through a model at their own pace or perhaps, in the case of preceptorships, over the period of time prescribed by the workplace for an orientation. Each setting needs to determine what works best for the purpose, time frame, and the resources set aside for the mentorship or preceptorship. The following six strategies suggested by Schwiebert (2000) are helpful to use for mentorship development:

1. Assess mentor strengths and networks, and determine how the mentee can fit into a network and gain from the mentor's strengths. Mentors who have not been mentored may not be aware of the importance of using their networks to assist the mentee. They also may be oblivious of their own strengths. It is often not the most famous professional who makes the most effective mentor.
2. Clarify expectations for the mentee and mentor. Both must articulate their expectations from the mentorship. Mentors should be sure not to base their goals for the mentee on their own achievements but on the mentee's potential.
3. Specific time needs to be scheduled for the mentor and mentee to meet regularly, and relationship boundaries should be adhered to.
4. Support, encouragement, and constructive feedback need to be given to the mentee at regular intervals. Allow time for the mentee to respond to the feedback, and then assist the mentee in developing solutions.
5. Ensure that the mentee is invited to informal gatherings, and assist the individual in becoming part of a peer network or facilitate the individual to become part of a new network.
6. Review with the mentee the importance of participating fully in the relationship. Otherwise, the mentorship will not be successful in accomplishing the mentee's goals. The mentee must ensure he or she is doing what the mentor has recommended unless they have mutually agreed on a change in the plan.

Typically, mentees are looking for who are direct with them, give positive and constructive feedback, are willing to share knowledge, are honest, are competent in their field, and are willing to let the mentee grow or become empowered. Preceptors can apply information from Schwiebert's (2000) six principles when developing an effective orientation program.

Zachary (2005) gives advice, worksheets, and exercises to assist in developing a mentoring program for any type of program and discipline. The following are her suggestions:

- Assess readiness to become a mentor
- Establish the mentor–mentee relationship
- Set appropriate goals
- Monitor progress and achievement
- Avoid common problems
- Conclude the mentoring relationship

Zachary also provides ideas for program development design to assist in developing a program for one's organization:

- Define the purpose
- Ensure viable support from top management
- Name the participants and the initiative
- Define the mentee pool
- Create the mentor pool
- Identify roles and responsibilities
- Develop the pairing protocol
- Build a mentor education and training program
- Identify ways to reward, recognize, and celebrate mentoring success
- Define management, oversight, and coordination
- Identify methods and procedures for tracking progress and providing for continuous improvement
- Plan the rollout or implementation
- Anticipate stumbling blocks and obstacles in the rollout process
- Plan the internal strategic communication campaign
- Anticipate mentoring casualties (affecting individual mentoring relationships)

Mentors, preceptors, and coaches need to be aware of cognitive learning styles, learning domains, and cultural competencies. Benner's Skill Acquisition Model (1984), commonly used for clinical ladder programs, is a useful conceptual framework for developing mentorship models. In fact, some precepting programs are developed around Benner's model, which depicts five stages that nurses experience as they develop through their careers: novice, advanced beginner, competent, proficient, and expert.

Generally, preceptors are in the competent through expert stages. Students are considered novices, and new graduates are advanced beginners. Due to the nursing shortage, there are not enough experts or proficient nurses to precept every novice. This is where the concept of multiple mentoring can be most effective. It allows novices and advanced beginners to seek out information from peers and competent nurses and then consult with proficient and expert nurses. Benner, Tanner, and Chesla (2009) found through their research that new nurses "know" which nurses are at what level very quickly after orientation, and so they know who to approach for particular needs. They also found it takes approximately 2 years for a novice or advanced beginner to advance to competent status. Thus, it would be prudent for a unit to offer mentoring or precepting support to all nurses with less than 2 years of experience. Zachary's (2005) perception of program design, which uses Benner's model, is appropriate here.

Training sessions need to include discussions of learning theories on how individuals learn. Strategies for various types of mentoring and coaching need to be discussed and determined for each type of learning experience (Harvard Business Essentials, 2004). Ideas from Dewey (1933), Rogers (1969), and Knowles, Holton, and Swanson (2005) are helpful for preceptors to review. Bloom's Taxonomy (L. Anderson, 1994) also should be addressed, so that mentors know how to discriminate among knowledge, comprehension, application, analysis, and synthesis when teaching and conducting evaluations. Examples of applying the Revised Bloom's Taxonomy in the clinical laboratory can be helpful for mentors and preceptors (Su, Osisek, & Starnes, 2005). Maslow's Hierarchy of Needs (1954) is important as it allows preceptors to review rationales for prioritization. Evaluation methods should be discussed, and formative and summative tools must be developed. Finally, legal and ethical issues should be integrated into the training of mentors and preceptors. Ethics must guide everyday nursing practice, including mentoring sessions that tend to deal with problems, conflicts, and issues, which may include ethical concerns (Hunink, van Leeuwen, Jansen, & Jochemsen, 2009).

Classic Mentoring Model

Nolinske (1995) describes a one-to-one mentoring model that identifies the mentor as an expert nurse. Nolinske also identifies a multiple mentor experience model that allows the mentee to have access to several experienced, supportive persons. This multiple model is comparable to the following description of the primary and secondary mentor model. A primary mentor presented a total commitment to the mentee, but a secondary mentor was more of a temporary role modeling experience or preceptorship on the side. Nolinske recommends the following five strategies to use for mentorship development:

- Determine the purpose for the mentorship
- Train mentors so they are aware of the goals of the program
- Orient mentees to the goals of the program
- Pair mentors and mentees, but let them set up their own mutually agreed-on rules. (The organization should set up general rules such as recommended duration, time, frequency of interaction, and an evaluation process for use by each pair.)
- Ensure that each is entering the mentoring relationship voluntarily and that no one is being coerced to mentor or be a mentee

These are several common steps in mentorship development. The literature suggests establishing a mentoring program as an effective way to recruit and retain employees (Cottrell, 2006; Hayes, 2005; Johnson & Ridley, 2008). Pontius (2001), a vice president of nursing at a large, urban hospital, recommends that RN mentors with the following qualifications be used: RNs with impeccable clinical skills, RNs who have been preceptors, full-time or part-time RNs, RNs not involved in any discipline process, and RNs approved by the director of the mentor program. This hospital developed the following responsibilities for each mentor:

- Mentor and coach a nursing student or nurse by discussing academic issues, clinical issues, ethical questions, and how to manage test anxiety
- Assume the leadership role in contacting the student or nurse and setting up a schedule with the student
- Establish a relationship that is comfortable for the student or nurse and is not intrusive

The goal is to support the person as he or she becomes more comfortable with the role of a nurse. It does not matter what clinical rotation the student is in for his or her nursing program. The mentor remains consistent. Once the student graduates, a survey is sent to the mentor and graduate or nurse to identify program outcomes. This program recommends hosting a reception during National Nurses Week to recognize nurses and showcase the mentoring program. This has been a successful advertising method. Outcomes have been evaluated as excellent for both the mentee and mentor, as well as cost-effective for the organization.

Pinkerton (2003) describes a similar mentoring program to assist new graduates and increase retention. Staff nurses interested in mentoring volunteer and are interviewed by the hospital's mentoring committee. An RN who is accepted by the committee signs an agreement to accomplish the assigned tasks of the mentor role. This is an 18-month commitment. The mentee then chooses a mentor from the identified list of mentors. There are three 6-month components of the mentorship, and so far, there has been no attrition. Of those completing the program (both the mentor and mentee), all have had extremely positive remarks regarding the educational growth of mentees, increased self-confidence of mentees and staff, and the increased retention on RNs.

Grindel (2003) offers many more specifics for setting up formal manager mentorship programs and says it is essential that there be a site mentorship coordinator with a support team. The team then develops a plan for the future manager and for the mentors. Included in the plan are mentor selection processes, implementation of the mentor-mentee relationship, a process for follow-up by the site coordinator, training of mentors and mentees, and evaluation of effectiveness of the partnership.

Multiple Mentoring Model

Those who are involved in a formal mentoring connection can still develop relationships with other mentors or be in a multiple mentoring process. In order to meet specific needs of new employees, some organizations set up formal multiple mentoring programs in which junior employees can search for mentors who can best assist them in a variety of areas. Burlew (1991) sets out the components of a multiple mentoring model:

- *Training mentor.* This mentor assists the new worker to adjust to the organizational climate. The person can be assigned or informally paired with the new worker.
- *Education mentor.* This mentor provides information on career advancement. He or she also focuses on training the mentee for a specific job, helping with developing strong support groups for

the mentee, making plans for the future, planning educational opportunities, and accessing new skills for advancement.

- *Development mentor.* This mentor helps the mentee develop his or her potential for the greatest growth and productivity for the organization. This mentor also helps the mentee accomplish self-actualization as described in Maslow's Hierarchy of Needs (1954).

This multiple mentoring model states that it covers all aspects of career advancement, psychosocial development, and role modeling. Actually, the mentee can have experiences with various mentors in each category in order to get the most effective mentoring. There are several advantages for mentees who are involved in a multiple mentoring process:

- Less wasted time looking for the perfect mentor
- Advice from a number of people
- Increased chance of diverse mentoring by gender or culture if desired
- Increased possibility to obtain mentoring from the most famous mentor in the work setting since this individual will be available to more than just one mentee

Similarly, the organization also benefits from this multiple mentoring process, as do the mentors, since they spend less time mentoring if they are involved with several mentees at the same time. Mentors also do not have to have sole responsibility for a mentee; if the mentee fails, there will be more than one mentor held accountable. The greatest disadvantage in a multiple mentoring model concerns the mentee who is not doing satisfactory work, gets lost then in the shuffle, and is not effectively mentored by any of the mentors available to him or her. Another method of multiple mentoring, speed mentoring, is similar to speed dating used for matchmaking. This model seemed successful for some inexperienced junior faculty who were able to interview for approximately 10 minutes with each of the volunteer mentors (senior faculty) and then choose among them if they felt any would be a potential mentor (Cook, Bahn, & Menaher, 2010).

Internships are generally for new graduates hired to work as entry-level staff nurses in an agency. Specialty units such as critical care units, labor and delivery units, emergency departments, operating rooms, and postanesthesia care units tend to have longer, more detailed content classes and one-on-one time with preceptors. Medical-surgical units have internships as well, and they tend to have limited classroom time and more one-on-one clinical precepted time for an average duration of 4 weeks. During this period, preceptees need to complete the competency-based orientation program for their designated unit.

Externships tend to be temporary summer employment for student nurses who are not internal to the hospital or home care system. The goal is to ultimately hire the best nursing students to work after their externships are completed. Many agencies offer these 12-week programs to recruit the students to work for them per diem during holidays, weekends, and vacations and then as full-time employees after graduation.

Peer Mentoring Model

As some people network constantly, this process of peer mentoring may be an informal adjunct for some people much of their lives. Often, peer mentoring develops within a cohort of new graduates, or between the current cadre of new graduates and the most recent new graduates who are now staff nurses with one year of experience. Peer mentoring is an excellent informal opportunity to form lasting networks that may endure over the course of a career. The relationships established tend to become stronger if the individuals have similar developmental stages. There are disadvantages to peer mentoring, such as confidentiality and competition. This becomes especially serious when individuals spend their time breaking the network's integrity in order to set others up to fail. When this type of behavior occurs, one or two mentees are generally the cause. Identifying them and asking them to resign from the group is appropriate. Clearly, their professional survival in the organization may be at stake, and they generally move from institution to institution.

Formal peer mentoring programs also exist in which new employees or incoming students are paired off with a "big sister or brother," a senior employee or older student. These programs are voluntary and depend on whether the younger person takes advantage of the assigned person. The quality of such pairings depends on how seriously the experienced individual takes his or her responsibility. Most organizations seem to use models of this type of mentoring assignment. They can also be found at websites such as the Nursing Net's mentoring project (www.nursingnet.org), which allows a registered nurse to ask for a mentor with specific criteria or allows the individual to select a mentor.

Mentoring Partnerships

Nickitas, Keida, Nokes, and Neville (2004) discuss using the service-learning approach in planning clinical practica for nursing administration students. They used the principles of partnership as described by Seifer (2002) to assist them in developing these rotations. Academia has used this model, in which a nursing student is paired up with a patient who was recently discharged or is in need of health teaching in the community who also is mentored by a counselor, nurse, or some other type of health care worker at a health care agency in the community. It is also used for nurses working in hospitals who are coming back for an advanced degree and may be paired with an undergraduate student in the same school of nursing. This partnering assists the RN, the nursing student, the health care agency recruitment initiative, and the school of nursing. With the nursing shortage, there probably will be more use of nursing students to extend nursing to needed individuals, and this can be delivered under a partnership program. In this way, the hospital, the nurses, the students, the school of nursing, and, most important, the patients will all enjoy a win-win situation.

An excellent example of partnering nursing students and RNs at health care agencies occurred with a college of nursing and two community hospitals. Students were told about the program and asked to volunteer to attend a luncheon to meet potential mentors. Nursing faculty were not involved in this partnership except for the initial announcements explaining the program. Rather, the program encourages mentors and mentees to interact at the luncheon and determine their own mentoring or shadowing relationship. What ensues is completely between the nurses and the students (McCadden, 2003). This two-way learning process generated outcomes including extremely satisfied nursing students and RN mentors feeling a growth of new nursing ideas from the students. Another school of nursing in the Midwestern United States developed a mentoring program for junior faculty and, as an incentive for senior faculty to mentor a new faculty, they offered a decreased teaching load (Blauvelt & Spath, 2008).

E-Mentoring

Just as schools of nursing are offering distance education programs and other work organizations are allowing some employees to work at their homes, so too professional organizations are creating national and regional databases of mentors and mentees in a variety of professions and then matching these individuals to create mentorships and coaching relationships. An example of an online mentoring program for nurses is shared by O'Keefe and Forrester (2009), whose hospital worked with an online mentoring program, Unleash Inc., to establish connections for one-to-one mentorships and networks of mentors to provide a multiple mentoring and peer mentoring program. They report some measurable outcomes of their online mentoring program including instant feedback, assistance in strategic thinking about one's career or an organizational issue, evaluative data that can be made available for performance reviews, conservation of paper, and increased ability to enhance staff knowledge and provide work related education. Another example of a successful electronic mentoring model was described by Miller, Devaney, Kelly, and Kuehn (2008) regarding their mentoring model of pairing up associate degree nurses with experienced public health nurses to teach public health in order to increase the number of nurses who could work in school and public health in rural areas of the Midwest.

Paper Mentorships

There are many nursing journals that give accounts of how a nurse mentored new staff, students, or peers. For example, Fox and Shephard (1998) emphasize the importance for mentors and mentees to share their experiences in the editorial column of the *Journal of Neuroscience Nursing*. This helps others to go out and develop mentorships by reading others' stories. Most of these accounts include some advice to the reader on how to and how not to do certain things related to career development and getting acclimated to a new job. One resource that is helpful for nurses to use in answering frequently asked questions regarding mentoring is *What Color Is Your Parachute?* (Bolles, 1999). Although paper mentoring is not traditional mentoring, it does serve to fulfill some needs of individuals new to an organization or career and can act as a supplement.

Multicultural Competence in Mentoring

That there is a separate component of this chapter on multicultural competence speaks to the nonintegration of cultural competency in the majority of mentoring models. Most preceptors are not of the same culture as their preceptee, so it is of utmost importance to have the preceptors trained in cultural competency. Actually, all nurses and health care workers should be trained, and there should be multiple strategies to heighten awareness. Some mentors and mentees may be from the same culture but have very different levels of cultural sensitivity. Coffman, Shellman, and Bernal (2004) suggest that nurses lack cultural self-efficacy, information, and experience with culturally diverse groups. Cultural stereotypes for Asian Americans, Hispanic Americans, and African Americans need to be discussed, and perhaps, doing role plays of some of these issues will increase awareness among preceptors so they do not show prejudice to their preceptees.

It is critically important for all nurses to be educated to identify and manage issues of culture in the work setting. With the diverse population today nurses need to be culturally aware. It is paramount that preceptors be taught about learning styles and the professional practice of nursing across various cultures. Frusti, Niesen, and Campion (2003) developed a mentoring model including all types of diversity, including gender, race, culture, disability, and religion, to increase awareness for health care staff. It is imperative that all nurses be aware of the career and educational resources available today in most health care settings. Leaders need to assess their organization's readiness to respond to diversity initiatives. The diversity competency model includes leadership commitment, structural links, organizational culture, and continuous measurements to assess the success of the mentorship from both the mentee and mentor's perspectives. Preceptees, especially nurses from other countries on travel contracts, need to be socialized to the culture of America and that of the health care agency. Characteristics of intercultural mentoring need to be shared with specific strategies to improve student cultural competency. Wroten and Waite (2009) suggest multiple strategies for reflecting diversity in mentoring programs and pairing people according to their background similarities. They share experiences in business and educational organizations regarding dilemmas that mentors and mentees face. They demonstrate how theory and practice must be integrated into a mentoring program in order to meet diverse needs. Green-Hernandez, Quinn, Deman-Vitale, Falkenstern, and Judge-Ellis (2004) offer insights into cultural diversity in primary care that are helpful for mentors and mentees in any setting. Zachary (2005) provides many cross-cultural mentoring strategies that can be revised and used in any work setting:

- Reflective listening
- Checking for understanding
- Maintaining cultural self-awareness

- Providing and receiving feedback
- Maintaining a global perspective
- Suspending judgment
- Maintaining emotional versatility
- Exercising cultural flexibility
- Creating culturally appropriate networking opportunities
- Modifying communication style to accommodate cultural differences
- Sensitivity to varying cultural perceptions to time, space, authority, and protocol

Johnson and Huwe (2003) believe there must be structured mentoring programs for minority group students, especially if the campus is predominantly one culture. Some of the components they suggest are assignment of a faculty mentor and peer adviser, entry into an established student support network, and planned workshops to prepare students for various aspects of the graduate program in which they are enrolled. They recognize that intentionally assigning mentee to mentor is not the traditional mentoring method but feel it is necessary to have culturally aware or similar matches as well as experienced mentors working with minority students. Boyd (2002) speaks to "mentoring at the margin," meaning that there are benefits and risks of working with students of marginalized status.

Nugent, Childs, Jones, and Cook (2004) developed the Mentorship Model for the Retention of Minority Students to assist students with academic support, self-development, financial support, and professional leadership development. Outcomes from using their model proved to be positive for retaining minority students and increasing their leadership skills.

PRECEPTING MODELS

Ulrich (2012) describes in her book, *Mastering Precepting: A Nurse's Handbook for Success*, methods to develop precepting programs for a variety of clinical units. She describes examples of precepting programs that would be appropriate for multiple types of clinical practice settings.

The precepting model is a one-on-one relationship in which the experienced nurse provides the preceptee with opportunities to practice, with supervision, working with the common patient types on the unit. This kind of mentorship is the most common process used in the hospital work setting to orient new nurses to units (Ullrich & Haffer,

2009). The preceptor facilitates opportunities for the new employee to practice each skill delineated on a unit-developed skill checklist plus whatever else a patient may present. A successful completion of skills and critical thinking situations allows the new nurse to complete orientation. Even after orientation, new nurses need coaching and further precepting when assigned to high-acuity, unstable patients with diseases they have not had any previous experience with, along with certain skills such as intravenous insertion, specific medication administration protocols, codes, and any unit-specific procedures such as chronic ambulatory peritoneal dialysis or ventilator management that is skill intensive. If the preceptee is a student, the focus will be on accomplishing course objectives, not on mastery of all of the unit-specific skills and challenges.

It is extremely challenging for a staff nurse who is already overloaded to precept a nursing student who is not well prepared. Matsumura, Callister, Palmer, Cox, and Larson (2004) used Grindel's *Contributions of Students to Clinical Agencies Tool* to study staff nurse perceptions of students (Grindel, Bateman, Patsdaughter, Babington, & Medici, 2001). The findings of the sample ($N = 108$, consisting of psychiatric and medical-surgical staff nurses) showed that staff nurses perceive definite benefits of having the students on their units as long as they are prepared and willing to help out with any task for any patient and not just their assigned one or two patients. Nurse faculty can have a strong impact on the success of students' rotations in any health care agency by providing them with an introduction to the unit and the organization to which they are assigned. Students need to have time to practice skills in the simulated laboratory, then advance to extended care facilities where they can become comfortable talking to and assisting patients with their activities of daily living, then to practicing total patient care and honing time management skills in subacute care facilities, then to hospitals, and finally to the patient's home. By gradually assuming more and more responsibility and having time to practice on less acutely ill patients initially, nursing students can gain confidence with their clinical, health teaching, and leadership and management skills prior to having rotations in hospitals and home care. Andrews and Wallis (1999) say that mentoring of students in England is the responsibility of bedside nurses and not nurse educators. Mentees need to take more responsibility for obtaining knowledge, skills, and experience themselves. With fewer and fewer resources being available in academia and clinical services, there is often little preparation of preceptors.

Models for preceptoring programs are set up for new graduates, senior and junior-year nursing students, and for RNs who are transitioning to new clinical areas and need retraining. A step or phase framework is not generally used. Rather, preceptorships are developed as one-on-one assignments in order to allow the preceptee time to gain specific experience. Often due to RN schedules, students have more than one preceptor to whom they are assigned to work with during a rotation. There is, however, more of a trend today to have a student follow the RN's schedule in order to provide preceptor consistency for the student. RNs orienting with a staff nurse preceptor generally have a consistent preceptor they are assigned to work on the shift they were hired for after completing approximately 1 to 2 days of general agency and unit orientation.

One nurse mentoring program was started due to low retention of RNs: 21 nurses had terminated their employment within 18 months of hire. The program was started with these underlying goals (Greene & Puetzer, 2002):

- Develop and maintain relationships between new and current staff
- Promote team building
- Guide novice nurses in the culture and environment of the new role
- Recognize and use clinical experts currently on staff. (A mentor was defined as an experienced and competent staff nurse who serves as a role model and resource person to an assigned new staff member. The mentor must commit to a 1-year relationship.)

The mentee was defined as a newly hired staff nurse participating in the orientation program. Due to time constraints and the orientation timetable, assigned pairings were used. A mentor was defined as a role model, a socializer, and an educator. As a role model, the mentor assists the mentee by example, that is, demonstrating how a competent staff nurse performs the job; as a socializer, the mentor integrates the mentee into the social culture of the unit and facility; as an educator, the mentor assists the mentee in planning his or her orientation. The mentee must be open to feedback, know his or her goals and work to accomplish them, have career commitment and competence, and demonstrate a strong self-identity and initiative. This model is developed in collaboration with the nursing process:

- *Assessment.* Make time to get to know each other, develop goals, and review the time frame and expectations. Review the competency behavior checklist.

- *Planning.* Choose assignments carefully to allow for goal achievement as well as long- and short-term planning.
- *Implementation.* Demonstrate knowledge through course work and use of current policy and the procedure book. Use a variety of methods so attitudes can be shaped through role playing, case study review, value clarification, and discussions. Practice skills are done in a simulation laboratory and also include critical thinking exercises.
- *Evaluation.* The preceptee must demonstrate evaluation skills with charting of data collection, analysis, planning, implementation, and outcome management.

Most say there must be incentives for all mentors but especially in nurse anesthesia, where the patient stakes are so high. Mentors should receive some of the following incentives: wage adjustment, flexibility of scheduling, and title recognition (Santos & Cox, 2002).

Hand and Thompson (2003) conducted a study of nurse anesthesia preceptors (N = 90) to determine their perceptions of mentoring and if they felt they were actually mentoring the students they precepted. The majority agreed that they were mentoring the students, felt the students perceived they were mentoring them, and valued mentoring the students. Seventy-nine percent had had mentors during their educational programs and felt they had had multiple mentors in their careers. Mentoring seemed to be confused with precepting in most cases, but a few had experienced a long-term mentoring relationship with either an anesthesiologist or nurse anesthetist. The authors question if it is feasible for every anesthesia student to have a mentor and suggest that it is the precepting that really counts. They advocate that faculty spend more time developing clinical preceptors to be more mentoring than trying to be a mentor to every student. In fact, they say it is important for the educators to be supportive to all but that is not feasible to be a mentor to every student. This finding is significant for all practicum-intensive graduate programs. A review of mentorship in academic medicine and anesthesia by Flexman and Gelb (2011) found a dearth of information in the literature on mentoring in anesthesia. One finding supported that self-pairing of senior anesthetists with junior anesthetists and students was more effective than assigned mentors and mentees. Recommendations by Flexman and Gelb include being more aware of availability of mentors, lack of time, gender and minority status differences, and generational differences.

Hayes (1998) discusses factors that increase self-efficacy as well as mentoring scores for nurse practitioner students. She found that nurse practitioner students do better with self-efficacy scores if they can choose their own mentor. This was particularly true if the student had a current relationship with the nurse practitioner. This information is particularly helpful for nurse practitioner program directors who may be having a difficult time obtaining preceptors. Acquiring preceptors is a labor-intensive process, so if outcomes are more positive if students obtain their own preceptors, it may be a win-win situation. Perhaps the preceptors may be more mentoring if they are approached by a student than a faculty member. The nurse practitioner directors can spend this time more effectively by teaching other aspects of the nurse practitioner role such as research, consultation, counseling, teaching, quality assurance, case management, and influencing health policy. Studies conducted with nurse practitioner students or even new nurse practitioners generally find that these health care providers do not get socialized into the multifaceted nurse practitioner role since the preceptor tends to be focused solely on direct patient care (Barker, 2006). Multiple mentoring models would best serve advanced practice nurses beginning new roles and students. Blankenbaker (2005) describes mentorships that have been successful for nurses in the military.

Role Modeling

Role modeling is a process by which a less experienced individual chooses a person he or she wishes to emulate. This is often done from afar, and the role model is not even aware of the other individual.

Shadowing Model

Shadowing is a process by which a less experienced individual shadows or follows an experienced individual through a component of the day's work. It is a type of precepting but it does not generally have a payment for the person shadowing nor is it usually rewarded by the work setting of the person being shadowed. The person shadowing is not expected to fulfill work at the workplace of the person being shadowed. The focus is strictly an observational experience. Prospective RN candidates sometimes choose to shadow a nurse for 4 hours or so prior to accepting a position on a unit. There are also many programs that link a person interested in a nursing career to shadow a nurse for a few hours. The nursing student shadowee has objectives for each shadowing experience that are mutually reviewed and agreed on with the person being shadowed. This is generally a process used with students, so there are also general goals for the shadowee to accomplish with the experience in order to complete the course objectives.

Grossman (2005) reports about senior students in their leadership and management rotations being assigned to shadow leaders in health care for a semester. Each was paired with an individual in one of the following areas (students did choose the area and when possible, although rarely, chose the mentor): patient advocacy, health education, research, quality improvement, health care policy, and hospital/home care administration. By engaging in supervised leadership activities such as negotiating conflicts, participating in collaborative decision making, assisting in health policy development and medical compliance assessments, and creating clinical and patient education protocols, students were able to practice leadership firsthand. Students' leadership development scores, as measured by the *Grossman and Valiga Leadership Characteristics and Skills Assessment* (Grossman & Valiga, 2009), were statistically significant and higher after the experience. Students kept logs and in their final assessments described their leadership growth experiences as stronger in that they could talk themselves through experiences they previously felt were too anxiety provoking to follow through on; felt more accountable for their work and this generated increased respect from the team and increased self-confidence for themselves. Additionally some felt they garnered the ability to be more enthusiastic about their ideas, more patient with the other staff, and able to delegate more tasks to nurse assistants.

Students demonstrated this growth after shadowing their mentor for a semester. The following themes were identified after reviewing three logs for each student:

- Growth over the semester, specifically regarding increased self-confidence with communication skills
- Greater interest in becoming politically astute and aware of the importance of the organizational culture of the mentor's agency
- Improved awareness of the benefits of partnering, collaborating, and networking
- Awareness of the importance of learning negotiation and conflict management skills

These themes are similar to what Glass (1998) identified as comprising the empowerment of nurses: raised consciousness, strong self-esteem, and political skills have an impact on the health care system. Nurses need to cultivate these skills to be change agents.

Mentees were excited about their mentors and shared descriptions such as getting more people involved in change, feeling the team valued their opinions, and feeling the mentor assisted them in gaining the ability to believe in oneself as very helpful outcomes of their experiences (Grossman, 2005).

It seems this mentorship helped to empower students to become more autonomous and accountable in their own right regarding leadership skills.

COACHING MODELS

Coaching does not involve the formality of a mentorship or preceptorship. It is advice given to others, generally on a regular basis but can be limited to even a one-time experience, in order to assist a less experienced individual in accomplishing a goal. The goals are not developed with the coach; they are strictly the learner's. In fact, the learner's goals may not even be known to the coach. Generally, the less experienced individual seeks counsel from a more experienced nurse, who then acts as a coach regarding troubleshooting complex equipment, analyzing laboratory or physical assessment data, or assisting the nurse to decide if a patient's condition is deteriorating. There are no data evaluating this process, nor does it tend to be sponsored through an organization. What transpires is generally spontaneous in that an inexperienced nurse seeks help from an experienced nurse. There are, however, coaching programs developing in clinical practice for nurses that are sponsored by the workplace. Coaching is, in essence, coming back, or at least it is in nursing. Many hospitals have set up support systems for the nursing staff using clinical resource nurses or clinical nurse specialists. These nurses do not have a patient assignment but instead are assigned to certain units on a specified shift to make rounds and assist nurses with their needs. Nurses also have the option of calling this individual to assist them with a challenging, unstable patient or help them with a procedure, admission, or transfer. Although mentoring is differentiated between coaching (a senior staff member teaches a skill to assigned junior staff in a limited time frame) and precepting (an assigned, seasoned staff member orients and trains a new employee for the first few weeks of being hired), there are many similarities. Certainly after precepting or coaching, it is possible for a mentoring bond to develop spontaneously and evolve over a longer period of time. In this way, the preceptor or coach shares the responsibility the mentor has to the mentee, which is to teach the mentee the ropes but also to share "the untold story, which is not always about the obvious workings of the job, but how the job really gets done." This "perpetual essence" of mentoring is the shaping of the mentee to create another mentor or preceptor or coach for the future (Fox & Shephard, 1998, p. 153).

VARIABLES TO ASSIST WITH MENTOR–MENTEE PAIRING

Campbell and Campbell (2009) suggest that teachers be hypervigilant about identifying their students prior or background knowledge and identify any misconceptions they may have prior to actually teaching class. This same process needs to be applied with mentors and mentees when they are determining who would be an appropriate mentor and even mentee for them. Any misconceptions regarding career path, networking in a specific profession, the organizational culture of a work setting, or the actual theoretical constructs which support one's ideas and content expertise in a specific area of knowledge all need to be analyzed when a mentee is deciding on whom to ask to be a mentor for them. The same is true for mentors who are requesting to mentor an individual–the mentor needs to understand what the mentee brings as background knowledge and experience, if the mentee harbors any misconceptions, and what the mentee's values are which are related to the areas that will be covered in the mentorship. It is significant for any misconceptions the mentee may have to be transparent to the mentor so the mentor does not waste time sharing ideas and experiences with someone who has preexisting notions that may bias them learning and growing. In fact, Campbell and Campbell (2009) stress that the language, class, culture, and ability of the mentee should be well identified by a teacher before engaging in class. So too, a nurse, prior to agreeing on a mentorship with someone, needs to be sure the mentor has similar language, class, culture, and ability prior to developing a mentorship. Wroten and Waite (2009) recommend that mentors and mentees be matched by similar backgrounds so that emotional and cultural support are provided to both the mentor and mentee. The National League for Nursing (2006) has a *Mentoring for Faculty Tool Kit* that shares multiple strategies for pairing mentors and mentees, and is available for use at www.nln.org/facultydevelopment/mentoring-Toolkit/index.htm. It has been pointed out that clinical teachers need a different skill set than clinical nurses and a clinically expert nurse cannot automatically be successful teaching in the clinical arena without some mentoring. Cangelosi, Crocker, and Sorrell (2009) paired clinicians with educators for a mentorship so that both would increase their knowledge and skill set.

Another method of pairing mentors and mentees in a mentorship was shared by Riley and Fearing (2009), who paired a nurse educator graduate student and a BSN student using mentoring as a student–centered teaching-learning strategy. This mentorship allowed for valuable learning for the mentees, who cited the mentors as crucial in assisting them with passing a nursing course successfully, and the graduate students also reported positive outcomes for their learning.

CONCLUSION

It seems that the ideal mentoring, precepting, and coaching models would have to be both informally and formally assigned with traditional mentoring connections. Multiple mentoring models appear to be the most appropriate option for new nurses in all areas of practice. The classic mentoring process is most appropriate for the doctoral student or new faculty member who needs long-term mentoring in order to be successful. Peer mentoring models are informal networks that assist all individuals to gain benefits. One-size mentoring programs do not exist. There needs to be individualization depending on the mentee's and organization's needs. More research is needed on how best to provide cultural competency in mentoring models, but it is true that mentors and mentees from the same cultural background are more effective than pairing people with different backgrounds. The idea of having several mentors in an individual's career seems to be most effective. Alliances with a mentor may develop in various ways over one's adult life, both professionally and personally. Effective mentoring increases productivity and adds to a more collegial relationship. Using strengths from individuals from all the generation groups seems to be advantageous for mentorships. The profession has a long road to go before the mentoring culture will be evident in all settings.

REFERENCES

Allen, R., Eby, L., & Lentz, E. (2006). Mentoring behaviors and mentorship quality associated with formal mentoring programs: Closing the gap between research and practice. *Journal of Applied Psychology, 91*, 567–568.

Allen, T., Eby, L., Poteet, M., & Lentz, E. (2004). Career benefits associated with mentoring for proteges: A meta analysis. *Journal of Applied Psychology, 89*, 127–139.

Anderson, L. (1994). *Bloom's taxonomy: A forty-year retrospective.* New York, NY: NSSE.

Andrews, M., & Wallis, M. (1999). Mentorship in nursing: A literature review. *Journal of Advanced Nursing, 29,* 201–207.

Barker, E. R. (2006). Mentoring- a complex relationship. *Journal of the American Academy of Nurse Practitioners, 18*(2), 56–61.

Benner, P. (1984). *From novice to expert: Excellence and power in clinical nursing practice.* Menlo Park, CA: Addison-Wesley.

Benner, P., Tanner, C., & Chesla, C. (2009). *Expertise in nursing practice: Caring, clinical judgment, and ethics* (2nd ed.). New York, NY: Springer.

Bennetts, C. (2000). The traditional mentor relationship and the well-being of creative individuals in school and work. *International Journal of Health Promotion and Education, 38,* 22–27.

Blankenbaker, S. (2005). Mentor training in a military nurse corps. *Journal for Nurses in Staff Development, 39,* 490–492.

Blauvelt, M. J., & Spath, M. L. (2008). Passing the torch: A faculty mentoring program at one school of nursing. *Nursing Education Perspectives, 29*(1), 29–33.

Bolles, R. (1999). *What color is your parachute?* Berkeley, CA: Ten Speed Press.

Bower, F. (2000). *Nurses taking the lead: Personal qualities of effective leadership.* Philadelphia, PA: W. B. Saunders.

Boyd, N. (2002). Mentoring dilemmas: Developmental relationships within multicultural organizations. *Journal of Occupational and Organizational Psychology, 75,* 123–126.

Brunetto, Y., Farr-Wharton, R., & Shacklock, K. (2012). Communication, training, well-being, and commitment across nurse generations. *Nursing Outlook, 60*(1), 7–15.

Burlew, L. (1991). Multiple mentor model: A conceptual framework. *Journal of Career Development, 17,* 213–221.

Byrne, M., & Keefe, M. (2003). A mentored experience (K01) in maternal–infant research. *Journal of Professional Nursing, 19,* 66–75.

Campbell, L. M., & Campbell, B. (2009). *Mindful learning: 101 proven strategies for student and teacher success.* Thousand Oaks, CA: Corwin Press.

Cangelosi, P. R., Crocker, S., & Sorrell, J. M. (2009). Expert to novice: Clinicians learning new roles as clinical nurse educators. *Nursing Education Perspectives, 30*(6), 367–371.

Cary, S. (2008). Mentoring generations today for tomorrow's leaders. *Nephrology Nursing Journal, 35*(2), 118–119.

Coffman, M., Shellman, J., & Bernal, H. (2004). An integrative review of American nurses' perceived cultural self-efficacy. *Journal of Nursing Scholarship, 36,* 180–185.

Cook, D. A., Bahn, R. S., & Menaher, R. (2010). Speed mentoring: An innovative method to facilitate mentoring relationships. *Medical Teacher, 32*(8), 692–694.

Cottrell, D. (2006). *Monday morning mentoring: Ten lessons to guide you up the ladder.* New York, NY: Harper Collins Publishers.

Dewey, J. (1933). *How we teach: A restatement of the relation of reflective thinking to the education process.* Boston, MA: Heath.

Ensher, E., & Murphy, S. (2005). *Power mentoring: How successful mentors and protégés get the most out of their relationships.* San Francisco, CA: John Wiley & Sons.

Flexman, A. M., & Gelb, A. W. (2011). Mentorship in anesthesia. *Current Opinion in Anesthesiology, 24,* 676–681.

Fox, S., & Shephard, T. (1998). The essence of mentoring. *Journal of Neuroscience Nursing, 30,* 1–3.

Frusti, D., Niesen, K., & Campion, J. (2003). Creating a culturally competent organization: Use of the diversity competency model. *Journal of Nursing Administration, 33,* 31–38.

George, D., Whitehouse, C., & Whitehouse, P. (2011). A model of intergenerativity: How the intergenerational school is bringing the generations together to foster collective wisdom and community health. *Journal of Intergenerational Relationships, 9*(4), 389–404.

Glass, N. (1998). Becoming de-silenced and reclaiming voice: Women nurses speak out. In I. Kelleher & P. McInerney (Eds.), *Nursing matters* (pp. 127–137). Melbourne, Australia: Harcourt Brace.

Green-Hernandez, C., Quinn, A., Deman-Vitale, S., Falkenstern, S., & Judge-Ellis, T. (2004). Making primary care culturally competent. *Nurse Practitioner, 29,* 49–55.

Greene, M., & Puetzer, M. (2002). The value of mentoring: A strategic approach to retention and recruitment. *Journal of Nursing Care Quality, 17,* 67–74.

Grindel, C. (2003). Mentoring managers. *Nephrology Nursing Journal, 30,* 517–522.

Grindel, C. G., Bateman, A. L., Patsdaughter, C. A., Babington, L. M., & Medici, G. (2001). Student contributions to clinical agencies: A comparison of adult health and psychiatric staff nurses' perceptions. *Nursing and Health Care Perspectives, 22,* 197–202.

Grossman, S. (2005). Developing leadership through shadowing a leader in health care. In H. Feldman & M. Greenberg (Eds.), *Educating nurses for leadership* (pp. 266–278). New York, NY: Springer.

Grossman, S., & Valiga, T. (2009). *The new leadership challenge: Creating the future of nursing* (3rd ed.). Philadelphia, PA: F. A. Davis.

Hand, R., & Thompson, E. (2003). Are we really mentoring our students? *American Association of Nurse Anesthesia Journal, 71,* 105–108.

Harvard Business Essentials. (2004). *Coaching and mentoring: How to develop top talent and achieve stronger performance.* Boston, MA: Harvard Business School Press.

Hayes, E. F. (1998). Mentoring and nurse practitioner student self-efficacy. *Western Journal of Nursing Research, 20,* 521–535.

Hayes, E. F. (2005). Approaches to mentoring: How to mentor and be mentored. *Journal of the American Academy of Nurse Practitioners, 17*(11), 442–445.

Hunink, D., van Leeuwen, R., Jansen, M., & Jochemsen, H. (2009). Moral issues in mentoring sessions. *Nursing Ethics, 16*(46), 487–498.

Hurley, C., & Snowden, S. (2008). Mentoring in times of change. *Nursing in Critical Care, 13*(5), 269–275.

Johnson, W., & Huwe, J. (2003). *Getting mentored: In graduate school.* Washington, DC: American Psychological Association.

Johnson, W., & Ridley, C. (2008). *The elements of mentoring* (2nd ed.). New York, NY: Palgrave MacMillan.

Knowles, M., Holton, E. F., & Swanson, R. A. (2005). *The adult learner: The definitive classic in adult education and human resource development.* St. Louis, MO: Elsevier.

Kram, K. (1983). Phases of the mentor relationship. *Academy of Management Journal, 26,* 608–625.

Kupperschmidt, B. R. (2006). Addressing multigenerational conflict: Mutual respect and carefronting as a strategy. *The Online Journal of Issues in Nursing, 11*(2). Manuscript 3. Retrieved from http://www.nursingworld. org/MainMenuCategories/ANAMarketplace/ANAPeriodicals/OJIN/ TableofContents/Volume112006/No2May06/tpc30_316075.html

Luna, G., & Cullen, D. (2000). *Empowering the faculty: Mentoring redirected and renewed.* Washington, DC: George Washington University Press.

Maslow, A. (1954). *Motivation and personality.* New York, NY: Harper & Row.

Matsumura, G., Callister, L., Palmer, S., Cox, A., & Larsen, L. (2004). Staff nurse perceptions of the contributions of students to clinical agencies. *Nursing Education Perspectives, 25,* 297–303.

McCadden, L. (2003). Perfect partnerships: Mentor program lets nursing students and professional learn from one another. *Advance for Nurses, New England, 9,* 23, 38.

Miller, L. C., Devaney, S. W., Kelly, G. L., & Kuehn, A. F. (2008). E-mentoring in public health nursing practice. *The Journal of Continuing Education in Nursing, 39*(9), 394–399.

National League for Nursing. (2006). *Mentoring faculty tool kit.* Retrieved from http://www.nln.org/facultydevelopment/mentoringToolkit/index.htm

Nickitas, D., Keida, R., Nokes, K., & Neville, S. (2004). Nurturing nursing future through nurse executive partnerships. *Nursing Economics, 22,* 258–263.

Nolinske, T. (1995). Multiple mentoring relationships facilitate learning during fieldwork. *American Journal of Occupational Therapy, 49,* 39–43.

Nugent, K., Childs, G., Jones, R., & Cook, P. (2004). A mentorship model for the retention of minority students. *Nursing Outlook, 52,* 89–94.

O'Keefe, T., & Forrester, D. A. (2009). A successful online mentoring program for nurses. *Nursing Administration Quarterly, 33*(3), 245–250.

Pinkerton, S. (2003). Mentoring new graduates. *Nursing Economics, 2,* 202–203.

Pitt-Catsouphe, M., & Smyer, M. (2007). *The twenty-first century multigenerational workplace* (Issue Brief No. 09). The Center on Aging and Work. Retrieved from http://www.bc.edu/aging and work

Pontius, C. (2001). Meant to be a mentor. *Nursing Management, 32,* 35.

Riley, M., & Fearing, A. D. (2009). Mentoring as a teaching-learning strategy in nursing. *MEDSURG Nursing, 18*(4), 228–233.

Rogers, C. (1969). *Freedom to learn: A view of what education might become.* New York, NY: C. E. Merrill.

Santos, S., & Cox, K. (2002). Generational tension among nurses. *American Journal of Nursing, 102*(1), 11.

Schwiebert, N. (2000). *Mentoring: Creating connected, empowered relationships.* Alexandria, VA: American Counseling Association.

Seifer, S. (2002). From placement site to partnership: The promise of service learning. *Journal of Nursing Education, 41,* 431–432.

Senge, P., Kleiner, A., Roberts, C., Ross, R., & Smith, B. (1994). *The fifth discipline fieldbook: Strategies and tools for building a learning organization.* New York, NY: Doubleday.

Senge, P., Scharmer, C., Jaworski, J., & Flowers, B. (2004). *Presence: Human purpose and the field of the future.* Cambridge, MA: Society for Organizational Learning.

Sherman, R. (2006). Leading a multigenerational nursing workforce: Issues, challenges and strategies. *The Online Journal of Issues in Nursing, 11*(2). Retrieved from http://www.medscape.com/viewarticle/536480

Stewart, D. W. (2006). Generational mentoring. *The Journal of Continuing Education in Nursing, 37*(3), 113–120.

Su, W., Osisek, P., & Starnes, B. (2005). Using the revised Bloom's taxonomy in the clinical laboratory: Learning, teaching, and assessing. *Nurse Educator, 30*, 117–122.

Ullrich, S., & Haffer, A. (2009). *Precepting in nursing: Developing an effective workforce.* Sudbury, MA: Jones & Bartlett Publishers.

Ulrich, B. (2012). *Mastering precepting: A nurse's handbook for success.* Indianapolis, IN: Sigma Theta Tau.

White, S. (2007). How to find and succeed as a mentor. *American Journal of Health System Pharmacy, 64*, 1258–1259.

Wilkes, Z. (2006). The student-mentor relationship: A review of the literature. *Nursing Standard, 20*(37), 42–47.

Wroten, S. J., & Waite, R. (2009). A call to action: Mentoring within the nursing profession—A wonderful gift to give and share. *Association of Black Nursing Faculty Journal, 20*(4), 106–108.

Zachary, L. (2005). *Creating a mentoring culture: The organization.* San Francisco, CA: Jossey-Bass.

Zachary, L. (2009). *The mentee's guide: Making mentoring work for you.* San Francisco, CA: Jossey-Bass.

5

The Mentor Perspective on How Best to Encourage Others

MENTORING, PRECEPTING, AND COACHING

Preceptors can role model leadership for new nurses and students and facilitate opportunities for them to practice leadership, just as they practice calibrating a pulmonary artery catheter, talking with a depressed patient, or interpreting a telemetry strip. Coaches facilitate others' understanding of themselves and their own abilities. Coaching is the process by which one person (the coach—the leader) helps followers understand that answers to questions or solutions to problems lie within themselves. Being able to role model and practice behaviors that assist individuals' adaptation to change is also helpful. This validates the importance of the mentorship process, either through mentoring, precepting, or coaching, and confirms that the emergence of leaders is quite likely to result from such connections. What nurses do in their lives every day produces a certain type of wisdom, and this wisdom will assist nurses to lead others.

Much regarding the future of the profession of nursing depends on those who are mentoring nurses—the preceptors, coaches, role models, and mentors. Some are people in authority, others are peers, some are nurses, and some are from other disciplines. But all are leaders, and they are cognizant that leadership is not a position or a skill but a relationship (Kouzes & Posner, 2011). Most have a great amount of wisdom to pass to others. Davis (2011) has good advice for mentors trying to encourage others. He feels individuals should follow his ten intangibles of effective leadership and also includes wisdom in this list. He suggests that mentors role model for their protégés the following:

1. Wisdom—seek out new knowledge in your field and find a mentor you trust. He also offers a *Wisdom Checklist* of 14 different qualities to use to assess a wise individual.

2. Will—go the extra mile and make sure you make a difference. Do not quit and use self-discipline to succeed. He suggests using *Hogan's Motives, Values & Preferences Inventory* (1996) which measures aesthetics, affiliation, altruism, commerce, hedonism, power, recognition, science, security, and tradition.
3. Executive maturity—do not get defensive, use humor, it is ok to loose sometimes, and it is most important to stay calm.
4. Integrity—this consists of a moral compass, being consistent with decision making, and trusting others.
5. Social judgment—observe the trends daily and assess and reassess. Be able to assess the people and the situation and then make a sound and fair decision.
6. Presence—you need to be able to command respect from the group you lead. Be charismatic by being friendly, knowledegable, and enthusiastic.
7. Self-insight—Have the insight into yourself to know what you need to do to improve since there is always something you can improve.
8. Self-efficacy—the underlying belief in a person's ability to accomplish their her or his goals.
9. Fortitude—consists of wisdom, temperance, justice, and courage.
10. Fallibility—Everyone makes mistakes but you need to identify them and take responsibility for them.

Sullivan (2004) reminds us that when discussing mentoring, the question is not, "What is it?" but rather, "What can it be?" Today, with such transitional times in health care, it is essential for mentors to:

• foster optimism and hope for the future
• be strong leaders who role model how nurses can advocate for themselves and the patients by recommending their ideas to the organization
• communicate that nurses can and do make a huge difference

Block (1996) recommends that it is best not to fragment one's life into compartments such as spiritual, private and personal, and work and professional. Rather, he suggests trying to live without always planning every step, following every good career and professional move, and not having to always be in control of those around us. In his book *Stewardship: Choosing Service Over Self-Interest*, he recommends that leaders not try to help mentees define their purpose and meaning, but rather to let them do this entirely themselves, even if they ask for help.

Block provides ways to find partnerships and be who you want to be, and suggests how to become and remain empowered.

This chapter describes methods for capturing the role of an effective mentor; delineates characteristics of effective mentors, preceptors, and coaches; describes examples of effective and ineffective mentoring; and identifies benefits for those who participate in some form of mentoring.

ROLE OF THE EFFECTIVE MENTOR, PRECEPTOR, AND COACH

Most significant to a successful mentorship is having an effective mentor who possesses some of the following characteristics: has excellent communication skills, is approachable and flexible, is willing to put time into the relationship to give frequent feedback, is passionate about mentoring, and has good connections to assist with the mentee's career success (Billings & Kowalski, 2008; Rose, 2003). It is helpful to acknowledge that some effective mentors informally mentor multiple individuals as part of their role as leaders and may or may not have the above-mentioned characteristics but still effectively facilitate mentees in enhancing their careers. These mentors can share their experiences with mentees, preceptees, and coachees and positively influence their careers. Others (Kram, 1983; Shea & Gianotti, 2009; Sinetar, 1998; Zachary, 2005) add that it is also vital for organizations to specifically identify their goals of the mentorship and for mentors and mentees to develop contracts that are mutually satisfying to the mentee, mentor, and the organization. The contract should build on the mentee's and mentor's strengths as well as both of their resources, taking into consideration any potential problems in obtaining resources to maximize the mentor–mentee relationship. A contract between a mentor and mentee should contain the specific time commitment, frequency of meeting, expected mentor role (coach, advisor, teacher), short- and long-term goals, and method of evaluation with target evaluation dates. The Center for Coaching and Mentoring (2011) provides an example of a contract that could be used by any mentor–mentee dyad as do many mentoring and coaching books.

Stone (2007) adds that mentors need to advocate for their mentees to attempt to maintain their motivation and also to keep aware of all potential opportunities that could be useful for mentees. These suggestions can assist mentors to do the following:

- *Gather information.* The mentor always needs to be assessing the mentee, without being unnecessarily interrogative, in order to be able to identify any deficiencies, confusion regarding the job, or problems. The mentor needs to redesign the contract plan to manage these concerns.

- *Listen.* It is imperative to hear all of the information and ask relevant questions when necessary. Be astute to nonverbal communications as well.
- *Be aware of the workplace milieu.* Know what the grassroots are talking about, correct any rumors, maintain a positive sense, and stay connected to the mentee.
- *Be knowledgeable of work.* Be competent with whatever work the mentee is involved in.
- *Evaluate.* Be able to give both positive and constructive feedback. Coach the mentee in finding solutions to problems in order to accomplish goals.

Bell (2002) proposes using the Surrendering/Accepting/Gifting/Extending (SAGE) Model for describing the role of a mentor:

- *Surrendering.* There is sometimes a need to level the playing field to foster more open discussion between mentor and mentee and to remove the power and authority from the mentoring relationship. Any anxiety that power creates should be eliminated in order to create an open environment.
- *Accepting.* Most frequently a mentor will have some degree of bias or preconceived judgments of the mentee. It is imperative that the mentor embraces the mentee for who the person really is so that open dialogue can transpire.
- *Gifting.* Mentors must be willing to share their passion for their work with the mentee. By advising and providing feedback, focus, and direction, mentors extend their passion for learning.
- *Extending.* Mentors need to push the mentee to stretch for the highest goals and constantly challenge the mentee to go beyond his or her expected goals.

Jonson (2008) and Dungy (2010) advise mentors to cultivate skills in facilitating, guiding, encouraging, coaching, managing conflict, problem solving, providing and receiving feedback, reflecting, building and maintaining relationships, and goal setting in order to fulfill the mentor role. Grossman and Valiga (2009) say what separates winning mentors from losing mentors is *leadership*. Other recommendations come from Gilley and Boughton (1996), who advocate 10 steps to create a successful mentoring relationship:

- Create a network
- Allow freedom
- Invest time wisely
- Be willing to give to receive
- Develop patience
- Actively listen to increase the effectiveness of the relationship
- Hopefully have chemistry with the mentee
- Establish relationship boundaries
- Create relationship reciprocity, and be aware the mentee may advance beyond you
- Develop synergy

Certainly having a network that a mentee can become part of will be extremely advantageous for accomplishing the mentee's goals and strengthening one's own connections. It is imperative to have a mentee with true potential in order to even want to invest any time in a relationship. By believing in the mentee and giving freedom for the mentee to follow his or her own ideas, mentors empower the mentees to be successful with their work. A mentor must have the patience not to interfere and allow the mentee to figure out issues. A good chemistry between mentor and mentee adds to the possibilities of having a reciprocal, synergistic, give-and-take relationship in which both mentor and mentee open doors for each other. Levinson, Darrow, Klein, Levinson, and McKee (1978) echo these recommendations. As the initial writers and researchers about mentoring, Levinson et al. identified the mentor's functions to include

- sponsoring entry and advancement for the mentee
- providing skills and knowledge
- guiding the mentee through complex occupational and social paths
- inculcating cultural and organizational values and customs

It is desirable for the mentor and mentee to share similar philosophies of work, have even-tempered personalities, be flexible so as to be successful in seizing opportunities when they present, and possess similar ideas regarding the balance of professional and personal life.

Mentors need to fuel the mentee's enthusiasm as well as coach this person to pursue his or her goals (Apgar, 2008; George, McLean, & Craig, 2008). Mentors know they will learn from new employees who come with a fresh knowledge base, energy, and, in some cases, their own networks from graduate school or previous employment. Good mentors also know that even mentors need mentoring, and they must continue to build and rely on lifelong contacts who share their expertise. They must have a genuine and overriding interest in the business of developing people. Mentors need to teach and role model how to network, develop outside partnerships, and prevent isolation or "becoming silos" with little connection to the outside world. By building from the inside out in organizations, shared governance facilitates employees to have more of a voice in the system and to include themselves more in developing outside connections. An effective mentor can role model anticipating what could happen before it happens (Watkins & Bazerman, 2003).

Good mentors know there is more than enough room for the mentor to participate in the mentee's work as long as they are not taking over or impinging on the mentee. Some mentors counsel their mentees to have two mentors: one in the same organization as the mentee and one outside the organization, to provide different perspectives about work environments. It is only with partnering with others, sometimes even with groups or individuals who do not appear to be strong contributors, that true growth and success will occur. By mentoring others, success will be accomplished. It really is not possible to succeed as an individual; we must go out and partner.

Other suggestions in the literature include not taking over mentee problems and trying to solve them and not giving advice and solutions. Mentors who do this will only enable their mentees and prevent them from becoming empowered. The *Ideal Mentor Scale* measures mentee's perceptions of their "ideal" mentor (Rose, 2003) and can help a mentee determine who would be an ideal mentor for them. Everyone needs to develop good communication skills in order to be sure their message is being received correctly. Gilley and Boughton (1996, p. 76) relate an interesting story regarding poor communication: The stewardess notes the right engine is on fire and calls the cockpit and tells the pilot, who quickly shuts off the right engine. The plane crashes and burns ... what happened? The stewardess and pilot were facing in different directions so that the stewardess's right side of the plane was the pilot's left side. This example is very effective in demonstrating how significant it is to be accurate and articulate clearly. Miscommunications do not often lead to a plane crash but can lead to multiple problems.

Lanser (2000) says a mentor must establish trust with the mentee to have a successful relationship. This is very true and is part of what Kouzes and Posner (2011) talk about when they say leaders must be credible. Their study included surveying 15,000 people, interpreting 400 case studies, and conducting 40 in-depth interviews regarding what constituents expect from leaders. They found the top four qualities leaders should possess: honesty, competence, forward looking, and inspiring. These four characteristics equal credibility. They suggest the three cornerstones of credibility: clarity, intensity, and unity. From this foundation Kouzes and Posner developed a framework of six methods to strengthen one's credibility. A mentor definitely needs to be credible in order to foster a favorable mentoring relationship. Kouzes and Posner advocate that mentor-leaders follow the Six Disciplines of Credibility:

- *Discovering yourself.* Review with yourself who you are. What do you stand for? What do you believe in? After establishing standards by which to live your life, it will be easier to make decisions and develop your character—that is, your credo, competence, and confidence.
- *Appreciating constituents.* Determine the values and desires of your constituents, and engage in dialogue with them. Be present, and listen to them. Always seek diversity of views, and look at the whole picture. This will make you more flexible.
- *Affirming shared values.* Determine a common ground for all to share. Unite people through a collaborative leadership style. Renew your community by having frequent forums on topics of interest to all.
- *Developing capacity.* Be sure to develop continuously the capacity of each constituent so that people are skilled to do successful work. Keep people informed, and encourage risks so that maximum learning and outcomes will transpire.
- *Serving a purpose.* Leaders must be other-serving, not self-serving. Demonstrate your commitment to the community.
- *Sustaining hope.* During transitional times especially, keep hope alive. This will lead to more challenging achievements as well as goal accomplishment.

Reardon (2004) discusses the language of negotiation and makes several recommendations for gaining this skill. Mentors can assist mentees to improve and expand on their negotiation skills by modeling how to frame issues, develop specific communication strategies, and engage in successful-cross cultural persuasion.

Many have said that the best way to be a good mentor is to have been a mentee. But the question that arises is, "Is this assuming that one had a good mentor?" Not necessarily. It is possible to learn to be a good mentor even though one had a poor mentor or even no mentor. So, mentees can actually gain valuable experience and leadership skills from observing a non-effective mentor. Most believe that mentoring can be taught or at least role modeled (Werner, 2002). A great amount of what makes a good mentor depends on the person's value system. For example, Werner, a retired nurse academician and hospital administrator, shares that she frequently used to ask candidates who were interviewing for positions or promotions, or prospective students, "Tell me about the very best nurse you have ever known," in order to determine the candidate's value system. She conversed with them regarding their previous mentoring and any role models they may have had in their past. She as to inquired how they viewed their accomplishments—solely as a result of their own hard work or due to collaborating with others. The answers revealed significant information about the person. Werner points out that it is not what the mentor sees, does, and says; it is more about who the mentor is. It is traits such as strength, courage, independence, and ability to see potential in others that make a mentor effective.

Cohen's (1999) workable model, the Mentoring Model of Active Learning, assists mentors in being most effective in the mentoring relationship. This model has six dimensions:

- *Relationship.* The mentor provides empathy, open-ended questions for dialogue, descriptive feedback, perception checks, and non-judgmental responses.
- *Informative.* The mentor assists the mentee to assess his or her job, review job history, require concrete answers, ask for solutions to problems, ensure accuracy, and rely on facts for decision making.
- *Facilitative.* The mentor helps the mentee expand on viewpoints, provide information, analyze decisions with multiple viewpoints, reinforce commitment to goal achievement, learn the basis for current pursuits, and review career options.
- *Confrontative.* The mentor assists the mentee with assessment of readiness, expression of concern for criticism, self-assessment of goals, proposed strategies for change, and belief in one's growth.
- *Mentor model.* The mentor role models for the mentee how to learn from difficulty, be motivated, and be committed to plan, while encouraging some risk taking and reinforcing mentee involvement in initiatives.
- *Employee vision.* The mentor introduces the mentee to considering new career training, clarifying skills, assessing options and

resources, being confident with a prospective plan for career development, and being committed to accomplishing his or her goals.

Cohen reinforces the fact that this model should be seen as dynamic and fluid, not just as a theoretical framework of a mentor–mentee relationship. He describes some conditions that should be used for this model to be most effective:

- *Planned sessions.* In order for meaningful transactions between the mentor and mentee to occur, there must be adequate time on a scheduled basis for the mentor and mentee to meet.
- *Holistic experience.* The mentor and mentee need to interact over an extended time frame and must be free to talk about anything that influences the mentee's growth.
- *Active participation.* The mentor must participate in the mentee's activities and be involved in both personal and professional development. The mentor helps the mentee in transitions through significant life and work events.
- *Ideal versus realistic perspective.* The mentor should be able to function in all six dimensions of mentoring, but it is realistic that some mentors will be able to assume only some of the dimensions. In this case, multiple mentors will be highly useful.

Mentors should have an entrepreneurial side, whereby they can encourage someone interested in doing something off the regular path to do so. The profession needs to empower nurses to use their creative ideas instead of giving them to the organization or physicians with whom they may have worked. What does "being an entrepreneur" mean? It can mean anything that nurses do not usually do. Some say it is time for more nurse practitioners to open their own practices. Nurses can learn how to start up and operate a business. Independent contracting and consulting by nurse practitioners could be a good cash-flow business. If the operating costs were kept low enough to offer low-cost-visit charges, a primary care clinic could be very entrepreneurial in this day of high-premium insurance policies. People could pay cash and have insurance only for catastrophic events, so they would not be paying for high-cost insurance. Perhaps the insurance business would need to be overhauled to allow this. But this process does not appear far from reality. Whatever the entrepreneurial idea is, an effective mentor could assist the mentee in researching all angles. The decision to become an entrepreneur must be the mentee's, not forced on him or her by the mentor.

Every mentor mentors a little differently. This is fine because it is important to realize that one size does not fit all when it comes to mentoring. Effective mentoring is something we should all learn more about. Sometimes, reading through an assessment such as those in *The Good Teacher Mentor: Setting the Standard for Support and Success* by Trubowitz and Robins (2003) is helpful. Fort (1995) offers a listing of 10 important mentoring rules that may also assist in improving the effectiveness of mentoring:

- Almost anyone can be a mentor; in fact, undergraduates can mentor underclassmen
- Identify what you can offer a mentee
- Discuss how much guidance is going to be necessary and how much you are willing to offer. Determine how professional and personal you want to be
- Give criticism as well as reinforcement
- Invite mentees to informal social activities whenever possible so they can network
- Praise your mentees' talents to your colleagues
- Give new colleagues help in obtaining resources
- Be honest if a mentee is taking too much time or not enough with goal accomplishment
- Realize you cannot mentor everyone or be all that someone needs
- Do not enable
- Mentors can be effective with mentees who are similar and different from themselves

Bally (2007) and Zachary (2005) say mentoring will be influenced by the organizational culture. Zachary stresses the importance of focusing on the person's "authentic character values," which are focusing on the individual, communication, accountability, and taking some responsibility for the whole, not just oneself, because these values will need to be supported by the organizational culture in order for the mentee to be satisfied and successful. Today, in our chaos driven lives, organizations are trying to develop innovative solutions to effectively manage the constant changes faced by health care systems. It is even more important than ever for nurses to have an effective mentor who can guide them in their careers, where they will most likely have to have more education, change positions more frequently, and gain new knowledge as well as technology expertise in order to survive this constantly changing environment of health care. Tetenbaum and Laurence (2011) explain how to lead in the 21st century using Heifetz' Theory of Leadership, which translates to the leader disturbing equilibrium, managing both technical and adaptive issues, and involving followers in the organization. Mentoring, coaching, and precepting are mechanisms that can assist nurses in leading health care organizations during these challenging times. An example of how a mentoring culture can assist Hispanic nursing students to develop their professional careers is the Juntos Podermos Program in South Texas; and this type of program can be adapted in multiple settings (Cantu & Rogers, 2007).

Sullivan (2004) suggests multiple strategies for best mentoring practices in chaotic organizations. A good mentor is a good leader, is credible, and commands respect. Mentors do not necessarily have to be in a position of authority, but they do have to have power and be politically astute. Being effective negotiators, excellent communicators, risk takers, change agents, creative thinkers, empowered, visionary, and culturally competent are all characteristics of good leaders that mentors must have. Mentoring models refer to mentors as also being good teachers, facilitators, and advisers, or coaches. The best mentors "bless" their students—that is, they call forth and affirm the mentee's life and career aspirations (Levinson et al., 1978).

EXAMPLES OF EFFECTIVE AND INEFFECTIVE MENTORING

Benefits of effective precepting and mentoring are discussed in an integrative literature review conducted by Omansky (2010), where nursing students and staff nurses were paired. There are multiple studies of mentor-mentee dyads of beginning staff nurses and senior nurses that increased retention in health care. Also, there are many mentoring/precepting/coaching models which explain how nurse mentors precept and coach their mentees in a mentorship. Additionally, there are many accounts of academic mentoring connections that have been instrumental in propelling junior faculty's careers, especially regarding research. Loue (2011) describes, via case studies, multidisciplinary health care workers involved in mentoring relationships and offers many effective strategies for mentors to use. A case study of effective mentoring follows:

Cindy was a first-year master's of science in nursing student and just happened to go to a brown bag lunch with a friend, who was majoring in psychiatric nursing. The chair of this track was talking about her research in nursing care delivery and asked if anyone was interested in working with her on a research project. This faculty member had recently been funded to study specific patient variables on two separate units, using different care modalities in a nearby hospital. Cindy volunteered and said she had experience as a staff nurse in the new care delivery mode. This was the beginning of a great mentorship that included both professional and personal development. The mentor guided Cindy through her thesis, two book chapters, and two journal articles, and she offered time to discuss other goals that Cindy had over the 2 years she was involved in her master's degree. Afterward, the mentor wrote recommendations for her, included Cindy in another research project, helped Cindy obtain funding in her doctoral program, and served as a sounding board through doctoral study. Having had this excellent mentoring, Cindy was fortunate enough to know it was imperative to get involved with a similar type of mentor in her new job as a faculty member, so she would be situated well for tenure and promotion.

A case study exemplifying an individual who could use some effective mentoring follows:

Harry was a new nurse manager at a large health center and had received the mentoring that is considered needed for successful transformation from clinical level IV and charge nurse to nurse manager. He had actually been a charge or assistant nurse manager on two different units in the institution over the past 3 years. He never had the luxury of shadowing an experienced nurse manager. He also never had the opportunity to work on receiving or delivering constructive feedback with a mentor. He was well liked and considered by management as someone who had the correct leadership style and experience to make an effective nurse manager. After 6 months, he resigned and said the reason was that he just could not give negative feedback every day. He was able to identify the unit's challenges and was well received by the staff and attending physicians, but what he found impossible was being able to communicate directly to staff members when negative outcomes surfaced. Later, he looked back and said he did not have the ability to word the feedback in a more positive fashion and so just blurted out what he felt, and then felt so guilty that he ended up apologizing to the staff member.

Harry did not have the self-esteem to feel confident in his evaluations or the emotional intelligence to have the understanding that he had good working relationships with his staff, and was expected to offer constructive criticism to the employees. He decided to become a nurse practitioner and chose a more solo versus team-oriented practice. However, he soon realized he was experiencing a similar communication pattern with his patients who were not following his recommendations for a change in diet, alcohol, exercise, or smoking.

Could an effective mentoring experience have helped Harry? It is part of the mentor's job to assist the mentee in recognizing patterns of behavior that need modification. Through shadowing his mentor in managing conflicts and giving constructive criticism, Harry could have learned strategies to alter his communication techniques with employees needing feedback.

Unproductive mentorships can be dysfunctional for several reasons. Often, though, it is because mentors are too authoritative and critical or mentees have poor communication or no accountability. Whatever the reason, some guidelines to review might be helpful to identify an unproductive mentorship so it can be either stopped or corrected. Johnson and Huwe (2003) suggest that mentors and mentees ask the following questions if their relationship seems problematic:

- Are the needs of one or both the mentor and mentee no longer being met?
- Are the costs of the relationship outweighing the benefits for one of the partners?
- Is either member experiencing distress due to the relationship?

Johnson and Huwe (2003) identified the most frequent problems that occur in dysfunctional mentorships and offer the following characteristics of mentor–mentee dysfunction:

Poor match	Mismatch regarding communication style, work ethic, or clinical focus
Incompetent	Lack of mentor competence in clinical field and research areas
Emotional instability	Poor emotional intelligence and relationship skills
Neglect from mentor	Mentor function not evident; little time offered to mentee; no attention spent on mentee
Conflict	Focus is negative and accusatory, and no solutions are offered to correct problems
Violation of boundaries	Confusion; discomfort with relationship
Exploitation	Mentor manipulates mentee for his or her own good
Unethical behavior	Mentor encourages fraud or plagiarism
Abandonment by mentor	Mentor dies, is ill, has a job change, or abandons the mentee
Mentee dysfunction	Mentee procrastinates or is overly dependent on mentor

CHARACTERISTICS OF EFFECTIVE MENTORS, PRECEPTORS, AND COACHES

Most mentors want to be good mentors whether they coach, precept, or mentor. They should first create and role model a healthier lifestyle that decreases stress and balances career and family. Certainly, this type of behavior may be a radical change for individuals who work in health care organizations that value a work schedule of 12-hour days. Perhaps it is time for leaders to make some big changes in the organizational culture in health care.

Zachary (2000) offers the Mentoring Skills Inventory for mentors to assess their preparation to mentor. She recommends that mentors acquire the following skills:

- Building and maintaining relationships
- Coaching
- Communicating
- Encouraging
- Facilitating
- Goal setting
- Guiding
- Managing conflict
- Problem solving
- Providing and receiving feedback
- Reflecting

Zachary (2005, p. 221) has also developed a Mentoring Skills Inventory (MSI) for mentoring coaches, which resembles the MSI for mentors and includes:

- Asking for feedback
- Brainstorming
- Brokering relationships
- Coaching (at multiple levels)
- Communicating
- Fostering accountability
- Goal setting
- Managing conflicts
- Mentoring
- Problem identification
- Providing feedback

Mentors and coaches can obtain practice in these areas by working with others who emulate these skills. Also, mentors who have had their own effective mentors can review experiences that they had with their mentors that involved these skills. Katzenbach (1996) talks about real change leaders (RCLs), who perhaps can be likened to nurses who are strong preceptors and mentors who seem to mentor everyone but tend not to be in the limelight. A 3-year study by Katzenbach and associates demonstrates that the make-or-break factor for success in organizations that are undergoing extensive change is the frontline person, not the chief executive officer or senior executives. He identifies several of the common characteristics that RCLs portray:

- Consistently committed to the "better way"
- Courageous and diligent in challenging the standards and authority figures
- Dedicated in fighting for what they really believe in
- Empowering of self and others
- Sincerely caring about people and the organization
- Not out to be recognized and in the limelight
- Excellent sense of humor

There is little literature regarding mentoring women by women, but Fort (1995), Helgesen and Johnson (2010), and Branson (2010) confirm that there is a mentoring gap, especially for women administrators. Fort believes it may be because women prefer to be mentored by women and there are fewer women in some disciplines who are at a point in their careers to be mentors. Also, many women believe they are not knowledgeable enough to be a mentor. Fort cites several myths about mentoring that may be helpful to review:

- *Myth:* Having a mentor is the only way to succeed. *Fact:* Mentoring is a factor for success but is not essential for it.
- *Myth:* Mentors should be older than mentees. *Fact:* Do not assume the older person should be the mentor in a relationship. Sometimes the more experienced person is younger.
- *Myth:* A classic relationship is the best way to mentor. *Fact:* Networking and multiple mentoring models may be more helpful than some mentors.
- *Myth:* Mentoring relationships must be long term to be truly useful. *Fact:* Significant mentoring can last over only a few days at a conference.

- *Myth:* A person can have only one mentor at a time. *Fact:* Multiple mentoring through various networks may be extremely effective.
- *Myth:* Mentoring is a one-way relationship, benefiting only the mentee. *Fact:* Mentors can gain large benefits from the mentee and the relationship.
- *Myth:* Mentees must be invited by their mentors. *Fact:* Mentees should actively seek mentors.
- *Myth:* When men mentor women, a sexual encounter is likely. *Fact:* Obviously this is not true but even with men mentoring men, there could be a sexual encounter.
- *Myth:* Men are better mentors for women. *Fact:* Studies reveal that women mentors are more likely to affirm, encourage, and give examples rather than directions. Male mentors were found to direct mentees more and be disappointed if mentees did not follow their direction.
- *Myth:* The mentor always knows best. *Fact:* No one person ever knows best.

Fort also offers some suggestions for all types of mentors in The (Woman) Mentor's 10 Commandments, which are similar to Zachary's Mentoring and Coaching Skills Inventories. Once again, Ellison and Scriber (2005) offer similar advice for women who mentor women.

Helgesen and Johnson (2010) and Helgesen (1990) share their findings about women who mentor and explore how their approaches differ from men's approaches to making decisions and priority setting. Based on a study of working with women leaders, Helgesen found that women are most interested in maintaining a more balanced life; that is, they want to be involved in their work and their family responsibilities. They view themselves as more than their images at work, and they see themselves at the center of things rather than at the top. Because of this, women create organizational structures that are not hierarchical. They see themselves as integrated in the whole system, which allows for more involvement with everyone in the organization. This information sheds light on how mentors should mentor women.

BENEFITS OF BEING A MENTOR, PRECEPTOR, OR COACH

There are countless benefits to mentoring, starting with the fact that mentors can increase their own power from mentees' performance and loyalty (Restifo & Yoder, 2004), and that some mentors can receive credit for their recertification by precepting a graduate student (Harrington, 2011).

In addition, bedside nurses can be promoted to the next clinical ladder by precepting, and a mentor can receive information for his or her own projects, as well as grassroot rumors and talk from the organization through the mentee and his or her contacts (Mullen & Noe, 1999). Gilley and Boughton (1996), Greggs-McQuilkin (2004), Ragins and Cotton (1999), and Kram (1983) add to the benefit list:

- Increased self-esteem
- Lifelong relationships in some cases
- Increased admiration by administration of your skills as mentor
- Increased leadership succession in the profession
- Psychological rewards of helping people
- Increased motivation and enthusiasm toward career
- Reinforcement that all of the work and sacrifice is worthwhile
- Generativity needs that can be completed

It is important to realize that mentors not only give but receive. Ensher and Murphy (2005) point out multiple ways for mentors to become part of an initiative or change that might have been originally developed for the mentee. Some nurse faculty have expertise in many facets of the faculty role and can greatly assist new faculty in obtaining tenure and promotion. However, many can learn new technology and be mentored by the junior faculty regarding grant funding or even become involved in new faculty's research initiatives and publications. Many of the newer faculty have been fortunate to have had mentoring in their doctoral programs and have been introduced into networks that far exceed what faculty received who graduated 10 or more years ago from doctoral programs. It is hoped that the more experienced faculty will be empowered enough and have enough self-esteem to realize that reciprocal mentoring with new faculty will offer everyone benefits.

CONCLUSION

There are successful people who never had a mentor and nevertheless mentor many and accomplish great things. Many nurses receive more mentoring in a 3-day conference span from collaborating and networking at the seminars than they do at their own institutions. All mentors are not effective at mentoring, and some do not have helping the mentee as their primary purpose. Being a mentor should be an option, and not all senior people should be considered potential mentors. Rather, these senior people can contribute to the organization in other ways.

It is more important to foster a mentoring culture in nursing so that more nurses can get connected to each other and to individuals in other disciplines. The organizational culture is also necessary to support the new mentees. Partnering with other agencies, collaborating whenever possible, and reciprocal mentoring are what the profession needs in order to advance itself. This chapter has suggested many strategies to provide best mentoring practices and reinforces the notion that mentorship with coaching and precepting must deal with the whole person.

Bolman and Deal (2001) provide a story of one man's search for soul and spirit using a mentor. The authors define *soul* as "personal and unique, grounded in depths of personal experience" (p. 9). They describe *spirit* as "transcendent and all embracing, it is the universal source, the oneness of all things" (p. 9). Their book is a powerful one for mentors to review because they explain how we all need to relearn how to lead with soul and spirit, and that soul, spirit, and faith belong at the heart of leadership. Nursing needs to have more mentoring for bedside nurses and for the members of professional organizations in order to foster a mentoring culture. Today there are mentoring relationships available for many advanced practice nurses, nurses in administration, nurses involved in leading the professional organizations, junior faculty, and doctoral students. Certainly, every mentor cannot mentor everyone or be all that anyone needs. This sage advice echoes what is currently going on in nursing with the encouragement of using the multiple mentoring model. Mentors need to use their time wisely, and it appears that co-mentoring and multiple mentoring models may facilitate this. Kram (1983) reminds mentors that they need to teach each mentee the skills of the position and coach the mentee along the journey to gain confidence in order to be effective.

REFERENCES

Apgar, D. (2008). *Relevance: Hitting your goals by knowing what matters.* San Francisco, CA: Jossey-Bass.

Bally, J. M. (2007). The role of nursing leadership in creating a mentoring culture in acute care environments. *Nursing Economic$, 25*(3), 143–148.

Bell, C. (2002). *Managers as mentors: Building partnerships for learning.* San Francisco, CA: Berrett-Koehler.

Billings, D. M., & Kowalski, K. (2008). Developing your career as a nurse educator: The importance of having (or being) a mentor. *The Journal of Continuing Education in Nursing, 39*(11), 490–491.

Block, P. (1996). *Stewardship: Choosing service over self-interest.* San Francisco, CA: Berrett-Koehler.

Bolman, L., & Deal, T. (2001). *Leading with soul: An uncommon journey of spirit.* San Francisco, CA: Jossey-Bass.

Branson, D. M. (2010). *The last male bastion: Gender and the CEO suite in America's public companies.* New York, NY: Routledge.

Cantu, A. G., & Rogers, N. M. (2007). Creating a mentoring and community culture in nursing. *Hispanic Health Care International, 5*(3), 124–127.

Center for Coaching and Mentoring. (2011). *Mentoring contract.* Retrieved from http://www.coachingandmentoring.com/Mentor/contract.htm

Cohen, N. (1999). *The manager's pocket guide to effective mentoring.* Amherst, MA: HRD.

Davis, R. A. (2011). *The intangibles of leadership.* San Francisco, CA: Jossey-Bass.

Dungy, T. (2010). *The mentor leader: Secrets to building people and teams that win consistently.* Carol Stream, IL: Tyndale House Publishers.

Ellison, E., & Scribner, T. (2005). *Women to women: Preparing yourself to mentor.* Birmingham, AL: New Hope Publishers.

Ensher, E. A., & Murphy, S. (2005). *Power mentoring: How successful mentors and protégés get the most out of their relationship.* San Francisco, CA: Jossey-Bass.

Fort, D. (Ed.). (1995). *A hand up: Women mentoring women in science.* Washington, DC: Association for Women in Science.

George, B., McLean, A., & Craig, N. (2008). *Finding your true north—A personal guide.* San Francisco, CA: Jossey-Bass.

Gilley, J., & Boughton, N. (1996). *Stop managing, start coaching.* Chicago, IL: Irwin.

Greggs-McQuilkin, D. (2004). Mentoring really matters: Motivate and mentor a colleague. *MEDSURG Nursing, 13,* 209–210.

Grossman, S., & Valiga, T. (2009). *The new leadership challenge: Creating a preferred future for nursing* (3rd ed.). Philadelphia, PA: F A Davis Company.

Harrington, S. (2011). Mentoring new nurse practitioners to accelerate their development as primary care providers: A literature review. *Journal of the American Academy of Nurse Practitioners, 23*(4), 168–174.

Helgesen, S. (1990). *The female advantage: Women's ways of leadership.* New York, NY: Doubleday Currency.

Helgesen, S., & Johnson, J. (2010). *The female vision: Women's real power at work.* San Francisco, CA: Berrett-Koehler.

Hogan, R., & Hogan, J. (1996). *Motives, Values & Preferences Inventory.* Retrieved from http://www.drbobhurley.com/pdf/MVPI_Manual_for_Elec_Copy.pdf

Johnson, W., & Huwe, J. (2003). *Getting mentored: In graduate school.* Washington, DC: American Psychological Association.

Jonson, K. F. (2008). *Being an effective mentor: How to help beginning teachers succeed* (2nd ed.). Thousand Oaks, CA: Corwin Press.

Katzenbach, J. (1996). *Real change leaders: How you can create growth and high performance at your company.* New York, NY: Three Rivers Press.

Kouzes, J., & Posner, B. (2011). *Credibility: How leaders gain and lose it, why people demand it* (2nd ed.). San Francisco, CA: Jossey-Bass.

Kram, K. (1983). Phases of the mentor relationship. *Academy of Management Journal, 26,* 608–625.

Lanser, E. (2000). Reaping the benefits of mentorship. *Healthcare Executive, 15,* 18–23.

Levinson, D., Darrow, C., Klein, E., Levinson, M., & McKee, B. (1978). *The seasons of a man's life.* New York, NY: Knopf.

Loue, S. (2011). *Mentoring: Health science professionals.* New York, NY: Springer.

Mullen, E., & Noe, R. (1999). The mentoring information exchange: When do mentors seek information from their protégés? *Journal of Organizational Behavior, 20,* 233–333.

Omansky, G. L. (2010). Staff nurses' experiences as preceptors and mentors: An integrative review. *Journal of Nursing Management, 18,* 697–703.

Ragins, B., & Cotton, J. (1999). Mentor functions and outcomes: A comparison of men and women in formal and informal mentoring relationships. *Journal of Applied Psychology, 84,* 529–550.

Reardon, K. (2004). *The skilled negotiator: Mastering the language of engagement.* San Francisco, CA: Jossey-Bass.

Restifo, V., & Yoder, L. (2004). Partnership: Making the most of mentoring. *Nursing Spectrum, 8,* 16–19.

Rose, G. L. (2003). Enhancement of mentor selection using the ideal mentor scale. *Research in Higher Education, 44*(4), 473–494.

Shea, G., & Gianotti, S. C. (2009). *Mentoring: Make it a mutually rewarding experience* (4th ed.). Menlo Park, CA: Crisp Learning.

Sinetar, M. (1998). *The mentor's spirit: Life lessons on leadership and the art of encouragement.* New York, NY: St. Martin's Press.

Stone, F. (2007). *Coaching, counseling, and mentoring: How to choose and use the right technique to boost employee performance* (2nd ed.). New York, NY: American Management Association.

Sullivan, C. (2004). *How to mentor in the midst of change* (2nd ed.). Alexandria, VA: Association for Supervision and Curriculum Development.

Tetenbaum, T., & Laurence, H. (2011). Leading in the chaos of the 21st century. *Journal of Leadership Studies, 4*(4), 41–49.

Trubowitz, S., & Robins, M. (2003). *The good teacher mentor: Setting the standard for support and success.* New York, NY: Teachers College Press.

Watkins, M., & Bazerman, M. (2003). Predictable surprises: The disasters you should have seen coming. *Harvard Business Review, 81,* 72–80.

Werner, J. (2002). Mentoring and its potential nursing role. *Creative Nursing Journal, 3,* 13–14.

Zachary, L. (2000). *The mentor's guide: Facilitating effective learning relationships.* San Francisco, CA: Jossey-Bass.

Zachary, L. (2005). *Creating a mentoring culture.* San Francisco, CA: John Wiley & Sons.

6

The Mentee Perspective on How Best to Become Empowered

WHY ONE NEEDS MENTORING

With the current explosion of knowledge, it is impossible for a nurse to know all there is to know about one area; rather, nurses need to work collaboratively to provide best practice. This is also true of mentors: no one mentor can provide everything a mentee needs to accomplish his or her goals and find self-empowerment. At the same time, while these goals are specific to mentees and the mentors, they should also reflect organizational and professional horizons.

Most would agree that the majority of people do not succeed strictly on their own without help from others. But there are people who say they have never been mentored or coached, and think they have reached the pinnacle of success solely on their own. It is important for nurses to review their careers and acknowledge those who have contributed to them. Although many nurses have not engaged in a classic mentor–mentee dyad, which at least some nurses may have wished to experience, it is most likely that faculty, researchers, and administrators have experienced some mentoring. By realizing the impact that various individuals have had on one's career, and perhaps on one's personal life, more nurses might extend themselves to encourage other nurses, or even offer to mentor someone. Being able to recognize others' influence indicates confidence in one's expertise and knowledge, and high self-esteem. Being able to credit others is a sign of self-empowerment. Indeed, many researchers (Daloz, 1999; Murray, 2001; Parks, 2000; Shea & Gianotti, 2009; Sinetar, 1998) note that those who have been mentored will most likely mentor others. Therefore, a large pool of potential mentors, coaches, and preceptors is available to nurse mentees looking for guidance about their careers.

Again, it is important for mentees to look for mentors, preceptors, role models, and coaches in order to foster more of a mentoring culture in nursing. Certainly, there are multiple ways to connect with a mentor, depending on what one is looking for. Self-education is also important. Reading articles, books, joining professional organizations, and participating in leadership and mentorship seminars at one's work setting, local university, via Internet with E-mentoring, or accessing learning modules such as the *Harvard Management* or *Leading & Motivating* module (Harvard Business Press, 2010) are all valuable activities. More to the point, this chapter describes why one needs mentoring, effective mentee relationships, ideas for choosing effective mentors, preceptors, or coaches, and the benefits and possible negatives of being in a mentoring relationship.

Developing an Effective Relationship for the Mentee

As we have seen, previous chapters explore how to set up and develop a mentorship, the characteristics that describe an effective mentor (Table 4.1) and mentee (Table 4.2), and how to maintain a successful mentorship or preceptorship. Certainly, a good deal of the perspectives offered will also influence the effectiveness of the relationship for the mentee.

Mentees should have interpersonal maturity, self-confidence, experience in managing stress, the ability to benefit from constructive feedback, and personal determination. Shea and Gianotti (2009), Luna and Cullen (2000), and Schweibert (2000) describe findings from their research that include identification of characteristics of effective mentees:

- *Emotional stability.* The person has a good sense of awareness of who he or she is. Others perceive the individual as self-confident and having a balanced life.
- *High sense of locus of control.* The individual is committed to making a difference and has a sense that his or her work will influence events.
- *Interest in learning.* The mentee is willing to learn from others and receive feedback on his or her work without being defensive.
- *Emotional intelligence.* The person can develop relationships easily with others.
- *Achievement focused.* The individual has hardiness, that is, a strong work ethic, and follows through with work.

Nurse educators and leaders should foster these characteristics in students and nurses so that more can benefit from being involved in a mentoring culture, participating in a network, partnering with others to share resources and talents, and being prepared to mentor others. Of course, there are always arrogant people who think they need no mentoring and there are those who receive expert mentoring but still cannot deliver any outcomes sought from the relationship. Is it the mentor's fault that the mentee did not accomplish his or her goals? Probably it is not. In most instances, it is the environment or the mentee's not accepting accountability for his or her commitments that mitigates a successful mentorship. It does seem that the most successful outcomes of mentorships are related to mentees' possessing characteristics, as previously listed, that can be acquired by working with a mentor-leader and developing personal leadership skills. A student nurse who began to acquire these skills would have an accelerated growth process as a new graduate nurse.

Suen and Chow (2001) described the perceptions of undergraduate nursing students on the effectiveness of their mentors—who were, in fact, preceptors. The findings demonstrate that students felt their preceptor treated them as guests on their units, did not welcome them as team members, and endured the absence of the kind of befriending they sought. In most instances as well, students felt that the preceptor did not fulfill their advisor role. On the positive side, the students expressed satisfaction about their preceptors as assistant, counselor, and guide.

Since the study is about preceptors, not classic mentors, the researchers understood why two functions—friendship and career advisement—were perceived as absent. The results of the study reaffirm the importance of mentors and mentees or preceptors and preceptees being told exactly what to expect prior to the initiation of the relationship. It also validates the need to differentiate between the classic mentor role and all of the other roles that are often referred to as *mentor*. Additionally, having a successful preceptorship is an outcome of having both the preceptor and preceptee fulfill their responsibilities. Preceptees need to read their patients' charts and be aware of their laboratory and image reports, study applicable pathophysiology and care so the preceptee will be prepared for their patient assignment, develop goals and specific objectives to focus on daily, and bring in relevant information or articles to share with their preceptor and the staff. In fact, preceptees should be motivated and inspiring to their preceptors (Happell, 2009), so they can facilitate cross learning for themselves and their preceptors.

Grossman (2007) emphasizes that leadership is a major component of being an effective mentor and that it is significant that the mentee develop leadership skills during her or his mentorship or coaching experience. Some examples of leadership skills that mentees can improve by working with an effective mentor include: their vision development, ability to lead in a constant chaotic environment, decision making regarding risk taking, communication skills, abilities to develop networks and partnerships, credibility, and followership (Grossman & Valiga, 2009). Mentees can gain valuable insight into enhancing their own leadership ability from informal relationships with a variety of mentor leaders over a life-long career if these leaders perceive mentoring as part of their leadership responsibilities. McCloughen, O'Brien, and Jackson (2011) share the results of their phenomenological study of 13 nurse leaders' experiences of mentorship, which reiterate the importance of experiential learning and informal mentoring.

An important skill that mentees need to embrace is uncertainty and the ability to respond flexibly in situations. New nurses need to have the ability to work in uncertain circumstances and make decisions. They have to have a skeleton plan that is focusing their day's work, but they also have to realize that anything can happen, so they need to be able to adjust readily. This correlates well to Benner's research that resulted in the Acquisition of Skill Model (Benner, Tanner, & Chesla, 2009). The less experienced nurse tends to be more task oriented and rigid, as well as more focused on the parts of a patient and not necessarily the whole patient. As novices gain more experience, it becomes easier for them to see more globally—that is, they can begin to see the whole patient. By observing more experienced nurses practice flexibility, manage uncertainty, and favorably react to change, mentees can gain confidence to practice these skills themselves.

Clampitt and DeKoch (2001) provide evidence that it is more efficient and rewarding to embrace uncertainty than to try to eliminate it. They describe that leaders know they can never know everything and that not knowing is quite legitimate. More of this type of thinking needs to be fostered so the morale of the organization will stay high and creative strategies to embrace change will occur. These authors developed the Working Climate Survey, which measures one's tendency to embrace uncertainty and provides insight into one's comfort with uncertainty and ambiguity. Clampitt and DeKoch recommend that mentees take the Working Climate Survey to understand how they view uncertainty. Their book, *Embracing Uncertainty: The Essence of Leadership*, presents this tool with interpretive guidelines and offers suggestions for being able to be less controlling and more flexible in meeting challenges.

Robinson (2009) shares the stories of successful people like Paul McCartney and how they found their inspiration from their own creativity and talents. Innovative ideas by Robinson suggest strategies to those who are searching for their passion. Mentees need to let go of their own limitations and bad habits and think more about their strengths, and they can often obtain assistance with this from their mentors. Often, it is these self-imposed barriers that curtail growth for individuals. By offering opportunities for nurses and students to shadow a nurse leader, they can learn how to take risks, manage conflict, negotiate for what is important to one's unit or position on an issue, and acquire countless other skills that will empower them to succeed in their careers. McLane (2005) presents a narrative on a day in the life of a manager that is helpful to students and nurses beginning their first clinical day on a unit. Shadowing gives them an opportunity to observe a staff nurse as well as to see how a unit operates prior to accepting a position on a unit. It would behoove every individual to take advantage of such an observational experience. Two resources that mentees can review to determine if they are ready for a mentorship include *The Mentee's Guide: Making Mentoring Work for You* (Zachary, 2009) and *Finding Your True North* by George, McLean, and Craig (2006). Both inventories are composed of questions regarding their perceptions of their own communication, work ethic, self-esteem, ability to receive feedback, goals for their future, and needs from a mentorship.

The profession of nursing benefits if each doctoral student has an opportunity to work in a classic mentoring relationship. Byrne and Keefe (2002) describe their experience working together with a National Institutes of Health grant in maternal-infant research. They analyzed personal reflections over the 4-year working period and concluded that the mentee primary investigator must be organized, focused, and have self-direction. They also found the mentor primary investigator must have generativity, altruism, and expertise to have a successful experience.

Albrecht (2006) describes several strategies that helps a mentee determine what one needs to get out of a mentoring relationship and describes the need for social intelligence. He goes on to say that without social intelligence an individual will not be able to successfully network or even communicate with others. His strategies would be helpful for mentees to review and employ when desiring entry into the "good ole girls and boys clubs" and with increasing their networks.

Multiple leaders (Miller, 2003; Schwiebert, 2000; Sullivan, 2004; Zachary, 2009) point out the benefits of mentoring regarding increased self-confidence with various skills and evolving increased self-esteem. They say being a mentee promotes self-development, which in turn has multiple positive influences on one's career trajectory as well as patient care. Dossey, Selanders, Beck, and Attewell (2005) share ideas on reaching for goals and following their visions in order to make a difference. They say nurses can influence the care of patients in an enormous way. *Ever Yours: Florence Nightingale: Selected Letters* is a collection of Nightingale's annual letters that she wrote to nurses a century ago. It also includes the infamous essay written in 1893, "Sick-Nursing and Health-Nursing," which, even one century ago, was citing the importance of nurses promoting health to prevent sickness.

Many nurses do not find a mentor unless they go to graduate school, become a midlevel manager, or are in some expanded role. It is nevertheless advantageous for every nurse to find a mentor who can offer leadership skills through coaching, role modeling, or precepting (Restifo & Yoder, 2004). The most likely way a staff nurse will become part of the mentoring culture is if he or she began as a student. Educators in associate and baccalaureate programs need to be involved in assisting students to make more mentoring connections. These students will benefit from preceptors and coaches who advise and role-model them along the way to becoming graduate nurses. Faculty must be part of the mentoring culture for these students. However, students must also go outside the college and look for other mentoring connections. There is a greater tendency today for faculty to get involved with graduate students rather than with undergraduates. This is due to the benefits faculty perceive they can receive from graduate students, such as assistance with their research or connections with a graduate's work setting. These types of reciprocal mentoring outcomes offer a more direct payback when it comes to career advancement and promotion. All new clinical staff have a preceptor in their first few weeks, but generally after completion of the orientation program, there is no further relationship. There may be communication between the newly hired staff and more experienced staff member if the new staff member initiates contact. So how can the mentee or preceptee forge ahead to keep or develop a support system? By encouraging the communication between one's faculty and preceptor, the mentee will develop a mentoring matrix. This matrix will gradually begin to evolve and bring in more connections. It takes time, thought, and some work for mentees to encourage their mentors to keep communication flowing. A mentee who recognizes the mentor's contributions during the relationship with kind words, a thank-you card, an e-mail or telephone call, or giving a small token of thanks will motivate the mentors to keep connected. These connections are paramount for the overall development of a mentoring culture in nursing.

Choosing Effective Mentors, Preceptors, and Coaches

Shea and Gianotti (2009) recommend that mentees try to learn multiple viewpoints from several people; learn all that is possible about an organization; network with others; practice skills with experienced people; and keep a record of the mentoring experiences. Mentees can make the most of their relationships by following some simple rules: articulate goals clearly with the mentor, become comfortable with the mentor, establish trust with the mentor, and be willing to be flexible (Shea & Gianotti, 2009). They further suggest that mentees be aware that mentors are looking for mentees interested in a formal mentoring program who are

- self-empowered
- not living in an extreme stressful environment
- practiced in conflict management
- ethical
- interested in improving communication skills
- caring
- practiced in team building
- expert in an area of content that has potential for funding
- trustworthy
- assertive

Grossman (2005) conducted focus groups with senior nursing students who had experienced a semester of shadowing a leader in health care. The students identified the following as characteristics for prospective mentors to possess:

- Commitment
- Willing to give frequent constructive feedback
- Collaborates with mentee to revise goals as mentorship evolves
- Perceives mentee's input as valuable
- Demonstrates respect for mentee in the organization
- Able to empower others and assist one to empower self
- Provides experiences so student is shadowing and not doing delegated assignments

- Demonstrates creative and effective problem solving and lets the mentee observe
- Demonstrates effective communication skills and lets the mentee observe
- Advocates for change and flexibility
- Shares hints on balancing professional and personal life

Knowing what to look for in a potential mentor is helpful. Oermann (2002) stresses the importance for new graduates to be open to listening and taking advice from experienced nurses in order to manage the challenges of working in the hospital. She recommends that mentees go out and find a mentor since mentors do not necessarily come to potential mentees. Oermann reinforces that finding a person to be a mentor will most likely not be the preceptor who was assigned during the new graduate's orientation. In addition, most individuals will need to seek out more long-term mentoring during their careers rather than think they will establish a mentor-mentee relationship during their educational program. Parks (2000) reminds us that mentoring communities are new forms of support that are developing for young adults. An example of a successful nursing community, which developed from a group of oncology nurses interested in developing an oncology certification exam and fostering oncology nursing best practices, depicts how a mentoring network for nurses was created to share their experiences regarding oncology nursing and connect nurses with other nurses (Rashleigh, Cordon, & Wong, 2011). Nurses can take advantage of this philosophy by networking with people outside health care as well. It seems that the person desiring mentoring needs to seek out people in their lives to be part of a network of encouragement for them. The 20- and 30-year-olds need to find time to network with their peers and families for support and encouragement. E-mentoring is an excellent vehicle for individuals to be mentored who may not have mentoring opportunities otherwise. There are mentoring programs that can be accessed via the Internet, such as Mentor.net.com and specific mentoring programs via state nursing association websites.

Benefits and Possible Negatives of Being a Mentee

Kanter (1993) feels mentees will benefit from a mentor with professional power by acquiring reflective power. This is evident in graduate education and should become more and more obvious as junior nursing faculty become federally funded due to their mentoring connections. It is crucial for nurses proceeding to academia to have powerful mentors who can assist them with this necessary component for success as a faculty member. So too, powerful mentors will assist nurse administrators to climb the ladder and obtain the coveted nurse executive positions in health care agencies. It would be beneficial for all aspiring to higher positions to read Kanter's book, *Men and Women of the Corporation: New Edition* (1993).

Mentoring theory proposes that relationships change over time (Kram, 1983, 1985). Kram's stages of the classic mentoring relationship can teach mentees what to anticipate, so they will be better prepared to maximize the benefits they can achieve from the relationship. There are four stages:

1. *Initiation.* The mentor and mentee have their first interaction with each other and try to emotionally connect. There is uncertainty during this first stage, so it is crucial for them to identify similarities and use these to connect. If the dyad can get over differences in this phase, they can proceed to a positive relationship.
2. *Cultivation.* A tremendous amount of career and psychosocial mentoring can occur during this stage. By attempting to shift toward a mutual exchange of resources and learning, the mentee will benefit the mentor. This in turn will motivate the mentor to make more connections for the mentee. When one of the dyad feels a need for change, this stage will end.
3. *Separation.* This is generally spontaneous and occurs when the mentee has increased autonomy. Some will stop all contacts, and others will proceed to stage 4.
4. *Redefinition.* This stage allows for whatever the mentor and mentee want. The mentee can gain the most by maintaining a collegial relationship with the mentor, or perhaps they have become friends.

Restifo and Yoder (2004) describe some of the common benefits of being mentored: obtaining advice for career advancement, learning new knowledge, gaining awareness of organizational culture, and learning multiple skills such as stress management, writing, teaching, and statistical analysis methods. Also, mentees gain a solid sense of ethics, networking opportunities, organizational savvy, and improved employability. There are multiple positive outcomes that are a product of effective mentoring relationships. Benefits for students who receive mentoring and precepting have been described.

Dennison (2010), Grossman (2009), Sims-Giddens, Helton, and Hope (2010), and Waddell and Dunn (2005) discuss the advantages of being involved in peer mentoring networks. All give good examples of how peer mentoring/coaching assists with the transfer of knowledge to clinical practice. They point out the benefits of being involved in a voluntary, nonevaluative, and mutually beneficial relationship. Sprengel and Job (2004) specifically cite how peer mentoring can decrease anxiety in beginning nursing students.

Another benefit of peer mentoring is that less faculty resources are used once a peer mentoring program is developed in a nursing program (Hunt & Ellison, 2010).

There are negative aspects to having a mentorship. This section refers to the classic mentoring relationship and not preceptorships. Eby, Butts, Lockwood, and Simon (2004) found that negative mentoring can be powerful in predicting a mentee's negative outcomes over and above positive mentoring. In fact, it is better to have no mentor than to have a negative one. Social exchange theory says that some relationships involve positive and negative experiences, whereas some are just positive or just negative or even fail to meet one's needs and are neutral but not damaging.

There is little research on negative mentoring, but one of the biggest negatives that mentees have experienced is mentors who take credit for the mentee's work. It is possible to have both a positive and negative mentor behavior from one mentor. The mentee will have to assess if working with the mentor to receive the positive benefits outweighs the negative ones. Some negative outcomes of a bad mentorship include a lack of networking with others; being associated with a mentor without integrity, which may cause others to view the mentee similarly; receiving little to no coaching or feedback; and having no exposure to the organization or profession. Realization of being involved in a bad relationship is the first step. Then the mentee needs to consult with peers to validate if his or her suspicions about what is happening with the mentor are accurate. If the mentee is involved with a faculty person, it may be difficult to terminate the mentorship; however, the mentee should seek advice from the faculty's chair or dean. Findings from research ($N = 84$ mentees) by Eby et al. (2004) warn mentees to be aware of potential negative mentoring experiences—for example:

- Mismatch of mentor and mentee regarding values, work styles, and personalities—the most frequently reported problem
- Mentors who neglect or intentionally exclude mentees from important meetings; these mentors are perceived as self-absorbed

- Manipulative behavior by the mentor, as when the mentor takes credit for the mentee's work or deliberately sabotages the mentee
- Mentors with poor communication skills
- Mentors with no specific nursing knowledge, clinical expertise, or research skills
- Mentors who have a negative attitude toward their work, the organization, or the mentee, or have personal problems

It is wise to go into a mentor relationship knowing what each expects to receive from the mentorship. Setting up a contract seems to be going too far; however, it may be important to avoid some of the pitfalls of negative mentorships. One would hope that only a few such relationships actually turn out negative. This optimism would put the odds in the mentee's favor that someone who is in the position to mentor others is reputable enough not to have negative motives. Mentees need to be proactive and assess if there are any negative motives (the mentor needs to be dominant, or has unwanted work to delegate, or needs to exert power, for example). Perhaps it would be more helpful to determine what the mentor's track record is with mentoring and communicate with previous mentees regarding their experiences. It would seem prudent for mentees not to go into mentorships blindly since it is a considerable commitment for doctoral students, as well as junior faculty. There is little research that identifies variables to successfully match mentors and mentees. Shea and Gianotti (2009) warns mentees not to make assumptions about expectations from the relationship that are incorrect. They have found that unsuccessful matches occur more often if there are cultural differences between the mentor and mentee.

CONCLUSION

Nurses need to be passionate about their work. How better to be motivated than by observing colleagues who are excited and successful with their aspirations? Everyone can remember a colleague who was the best and at the top of his or her career but never moved on to conquer more mountains. For some reason, they felt stuck. Others who were movers and shakers grew tired of the status quo work setting and joined more ambitious institutions. As some work environments get more toxic, employees lose their self-esteem and self-empowerment, and become one of the losers. Donald Trump says on his television show, *The Apprentice*, that he has learned over and over that "one who works with losers will eventually become a loser." This seems to be true. Mentees who belong to mentoring connections will be less likely to fall into a loser environment, and they will have the support and strength of their mentoring network to pull themselves out. Mentees need to realize they are not entitled to be winners but have to work hard to achieve success. Mentees need to take some risks, work hard to connect with mentors, and accept change to be involved in peer and multiple mentoring networks. By improving their leadership skills through mentoring, mentees will be able to help themselves as well as the profession. Parks (2000) recommends that it is more important than ever before to assist the new generation in pursuing their dreams rather than focusing on self-interest. Mentors need to role-model well today in order to influence the future professional nurses.

REFERENCES

Albrecht, K. (2006). *Social intelligence: The new science of success.* San Francisco, CA: Jossey-Bass.

Benner, P., Tanner, C., & Chesla, C. (2009). *Expertise in nursing practice: Caring, clinical judgment and ethics* (2nd ed.). New York, NY: Springer.

Byrne, M., & Keefe, M. (2002). Building research competence in nursing through mentoring. *Journal of Nursing Scholarship, 34,* 391–396.

Clampitt, P., & DeKoch, R. (2001). *Embracing uncertainty: The essence of leadership.* Armonk, NY: M. E. Sharpe.

Daloz, L. (1999). *Mentor: Guiding the journey of adult learners* (2nd ed.). San Francisco, CA: Jossey-Bass.

Dennison, S. (2010). Peer mentoring: Untapped potential. *Journal of Nursing Education, 49*(6), 340–342.

Dossey, B., Selanders, L., Beck, D. M., & Attewell, A. (2005). *Florence Nightingale today: Healing leadership global action.* Washington, DC: American Nurses Association.

Eby, L., Butts, M., Lockwood, A., & Simon, S. (2004). Protégés' negative mentoring experiences: Construct development and nomological validation. *Personnel Psychology, 57,* 411–448.

George, B., McLean, A., & Craig, N. (2006). *Finding your true north—A personal guide.* San Francisco, CA: Jossey–Bass.

Grossman, S. (2005). Developing leadership through shadowing a leader in health care. In H. Feldman & M. Greenberg (Eds.), *Educating for leadership* (pp. 266–278). New York, NY: Springer.

Grossman, S. (2007). Assisting critical care nurses in acquiring leadership skills. *Dimensions of Critical Care Nursing, 26*(2), 57–65.

Grossman, S. (2009). Peering: The essence of collaborative mentoring in critical care. *Dimensions in Critical Care Nursing, 28*(2), 72–75.

Grossman, S., & Valiga, T. (2009). *The new leadership challenge: Creating the future of nursing* (3rd ed.). Philadelphia, PA: F. A. Davis.

Happell, B. (2009). A model of preceptorship in nursing: Reflecting the complex functions of the role. *Nursing Education Perspectives, 30*(6), 372–376.

Harvard Business Press. (2010). Harvard managementoring module— *Leading & motivating.* Retrieved from http://hbr.org/product/baynote/an/6789X-HTM-ENG?referral=00505

Hunt, C. W., & Ellison, K. J. (2010). Enhancing faculty resources through peer mentoring. *Nurse Educator, 35*(5), 192–196.

Kanter, R. (1993). *Men and women of the corporation: New edition.* New York, NY: Basic Books.

Kram, K. (1983). Phases of the mentor relationship. *Academy of Management Journal, 26,* 608–625.

Kram, K. (1985). Mentoring in the workplace. In D. Hall (Ed.), *Career development in organizations* (pp. 160–201). San Francisco, CA: Jossey-Bass.

Luna, G., & Cullen, D. (2000). *Empowering the faculty: Mentoring redirected and renewed.* Washington, DC: George Washington University Press.

McCloughen, A., O'Brien, L. & Jackson, D. (2011). Nurse leader mentor as a mode of being: Findings from an Australian hermeneutic phenomenological study. *Journal of Nursing Scholarship, 43*(1), 97–104.

McLane, S. (2005). A day in the life of a manager: Incorporating leadership, management, and role modeling. *Oncology Nursing Forum, 32,* 23–25.

Miller, T. (2003). *Building and managing a career in nursing.* Indianapolis, IN: Sigma Theta Tau International.

Murray, M. (2001). *Beyond the myths and magic of mentoring: How to facilitate an effective mentoring process* (2nd ed.). San Francisco, CA: Jossey-Bass.

Oermann, M. (2002). Stresses and challenges for new graduates in hospitals. *Nurse Education Today, 22,* 225–230.

Parks, S. D. (2000). *Big questions, worthy dreams: Mentoring young adults in their search for meaning, purpose, and faith.* San Francisco, CA: Jossey-Bass.

Rashleigh, L., Cordon, C., & Wong, J. (2011). Creating opportunities to support one nursing practice: Surviving and thriving. *Canadian Nursing Oncology Journal, 21*(1), 7–10.

Restifo, V., & Yoder, L. (2004). Partnership: Making the most of mentoring. *Nursing Spectrum, 8,* 15–19.

Robinson, K. (2009). *The element: How finding your passion changes everything.* New York, NY: Penguin Group.

Schwiebert, V. (2000). *Mentoring: Creating connected, empowered relationships.* Alexandria, VA: American Counseling Association.

Shea, G. F., & Gianotti, S. C. (2009). *Mentoring: Make it a mutually rewarding experience* (4th ed.). Menlo Park, CA: Crisp Publications.

Sims-Giddens, S., Helton, C., & Hope, C. (2010). Student peer mentoring in a community-based nursing clinical experience. *Nursing Education Perspectives, 31*(1), 23–27.

Sinetar, M. (1998). *The mentor's spirit: Life lessons on leadership and the art of encouragement.* New York, NY: St. Martin's Press.

Sprengel, A. D., & Job, L. (2004). Reducing student anxiety by using clinical peer mentoring with beginning nursing students. *Nurse Educator, 29,*
246–250.

Suen, L., & Chow, F. (2001). Students' perceptions of the effectiveness of the
effectiveness of mentors in an undergraduate nursing programme in Hong
Kong. *Journal of Advanced Nursing, 36,* 505–511.

Sullivan, C. (2004). *How to mentor in the midst of change* (2nd ed.). New York,
NY: Association for Supervision and Curriculum Development.

Waddell, D., & Dunn, N. (2005). Peer coaching: The next step in staff development. *Journal of Continuing Education in Nursing, 36,* 84–89.

Zachary, L. (2009). *The mentee's guide: Making mentoring work for you.* San
Francisco, CA: Jossey-Bass.

7

Need for Evaluation of Mentoring

The Institute of Medicine (2010) strongly suggests the use of residency programs and mentorships for health care professionals. Residency programs, which involve effective mentoring, precepting, and coaching, are instrumental in developing similar programs for RNs and APRNs. Since the literature has demonstrated that mentorships, preceptor–preceptee programs, and coaching have influenced nurse retention and job satisfaction favorably, it is important to identify what program components are correlated with success. The work environment is crucial here. Beecroft, Dorey, and Wenten (2008) have found alarming new graduate turnover rates in many hospitals; between 35% and 65% during the first year of employment due specifically to unhealthy work environments. The lack of healthy work environments, along with scarcity of mentoring and precepting, also seems to be related to poor staff retention and job satisfaction.

This chapter thus discusses several pertinent issues: the current lack of measurement of mentoring outcomes, some professional and personal outcomes that relate to mentoring, leadership variables related to mentoring, strategies to measure outcomes of mentoring for the profession, the organization, patient consumers, mentors, and mentees, and examples of measuring mentoring outcomes.

LACK OF MEASUREMENT OF MENTORING OUTCOMES

Documented results on the effects of mentoring in many areas of health care and nursing are clearly lacking. Most mentoring programs or internship relationships are evaluated, if at all, with qualitative open-ended questions regarding mentor and mentee perceptions of the experience. Commonly thought, expected results of mentoring are clear: mentors enable mentees to accomplish goals more quickly than without mentoring, and staff retention increases. The ultimate goal of mentoring is for mentees to become professionally socialized (Bandura, 1977).

Precepting programs and other university–hospital partnerships generally measure their success by the number of nurses recruited and retained by the health care agency sponsoring the preceptorship. Student preceptorships and shadowing programs are measured by collecting student perceptions of their experiences, preceptors' perceptions of student performance, and possibly student critical thinking scores or some other tangible outcome that is evaluated before and after the preceptorship. More outcome studies on mentoring are needed, especially those that measure mentee critical thinking, clinical decision making, leadership development, and how having been a mentee or mentor impacts patient care. Research findings describing how nurse acquisition of competency is correlated to progression on Benner's (1984) novice to expert continuum (Nedd, Nash, Galindo-Ciocon, & Belgrave, 2006) are available. Perhaps studying how mentoring/precepting/coaching may impact a nurse along Benner's continuum of different skill levels would be helpful in knowing what mentoring method might be best to employ. There is an enormous need for more outcome measurements to document the efficacy of all mentoring programs.

More than three decades ago, Levinson et al. (1978) were the first educators to study mentoring outcomes. Their findings include the importance of the mentor's believing in the mentee, sharing parts of the mentee's dream, and giving the dream his or her blessing. By doing this, they feel it helped to "define the mentee's newly emerging self" (p. 98). This "blessing" from a mentor to a mentee does convey a certain caring and genuine feeling for the mentee by the mentor and has been identified as significant for effective mentorships (Wagner, 2008). For its part, the psychosocial theory of development (Erikson, 1963) suggests that the final stage of generativity correlates with the concept of mentoring because it allows all who have a concern for improving the world to participate by mentoring younger generations. Luna and Cullen (2000) suggest that the dyad framework fits well in academia, where senior faculty mentor junior faculty to develop younger colleagues' talent and, at the same time, promote the department and university. Essentially, generativity is the foundation of a senior mentor/preceptor/coach as the individual facilitates learning for the new generation (Cary, 2008; Luna & Cullen, 2000).

Kram believes that mentees (in academia and business) can advance more quickly if multiple mentors are involved with a mentee. It is common knowledge that the majority of faculty who have had mentors are more productive in obtaining competitive grants, leading professional organizations, and publishing more books and refereed jou. articles. Kram also advocates for research on the mentoring relationship in all of its stages through longitudinal studies (Kram, 1985).

Although there are multiple studies of mentoring in educational settings, many lack any experimental design, use self-reported responses, have used little to no psychometrically backed tools, and do not differentiate between informal and formal mentoring (Allen & Eby, 2004; Allen, Eby, O'Brien, & Lentz, 2008). Nonetheless, the mentoring research in education, which adds significantly to the body of mentoring literature, supports the need to gather all perspectives and in multiple disciplines.

PROFESSIONAL VERSUS PERSONAL OUTCOMES OF MENTORING

Professional Outcomes

It would be helpful to assess the variables that affect a nurse's ability to be a successful mentor (such as clinical experience, education, and type of nursing the mentorship is focusing on, whether clinical, administrative, or educational). One would also assume that some of these variables come from an operational definition of mentoring and include the following: length of the mentoring relationship, whether the mentorship was informal or formally assigned, and the organizational culture in which the mentor and mentee worked. Professional or career mentoring is generally based solely on how the relationship will assist the individual and/or the work organization. Kram (1985) sees career mentoring more specifically as part of a mentoring relationship that refers to the mentee's career through sponsorship, visibility, coaching, protection, and challenging assignments. Multiple demographic or personal variables are often not included in these studies. In nursing, professional outcomes of mentoring can include a variety of achievements such as: certification in one's area of specialty; passing the NCLEX exam; becoming an Advanced Practice Registered Nurse; promotion to the highest clinical staff nurse position; obtaining grant funding; achieving a top administrative position in practice or academia; election to lead a national or international professional organization; appointment to a prestigious board; or selection as an expert in one's area of expertise in nursing or health care.

Allen et al. (2008) conducted a literature review of mentoring relationships in the workplace and found 207 different studies since 2006. They also determined that the most common journal to publish workplace mentoring research was the *Journal of Vocational Behavior*. In agreement with the Allen et al. (2008) study of the state of mentoring research in work settings, nursing needs to have more studies in the following categories that would specifically focus on professional mentoring:

1. Outcome research—specific results of mentorships
2. Predictor research—findings indicating certain independent variables were predictive of how a mentor or mentee behaved or scored regarding an aspect of mentoring
3. Predictor/Outcome research—both antecedents and results of mentoring
4. Measurement/Construct research—study focuses on a mentoring construct or a tool to measure some type of mentoring
5. Research review—a literature review
6. Theory development research—a theoretical framework is developed and studied

The profession of nursing has several definitions of mentoring. Most feel precepting is reserved for the orientation of new staff or the pairing of an experienced and inexperienced staff member when having an inservice on a specific type of equipment or new nursing procedure. The coaching relationship is considered a short-term, one-on-one, and generally, paid connection. So until the mentoring concept is clearly defined and accepted as standard, many studies will generate new information about mentoring specific to that author's own definition of the term, mentoring. Quantitative and qualitative studies are needed.

Personal Outcomes

The literature does not always provide information on the personal/psychosocial background (gender, age, culture, marital status, socioeconomic level, or financial ability) of mentors and mentees along with the above-mentioned career mentoring variables. Evidence supports that these variables would impact the mentoring relationship and should also be studied. Kram (1985) further defines psychosocial variables as including the mentee's sense of self-image, which she describes as involving components of friendship, counseling, acceptance, and confirmation.

LEADERSHIP VARIABLES RELATED TO MENTORING

Preceptors who are authentic leaders, meaning they believe that people wish to be inspired, were well received by their preceptees because the new nurses felt more engaged and had higher satisfaction with their jobs (Giallonardo, Wong, & Iwasiw, 2010). Authentic leaders increase followers' empowerment of themselves by identifying with the leader and organization that facilitates hope, trust, and an optimistic viewpoint (Avolio, Gardner, Walumbwa, Luthan, & May, 2004). An *Authentic Leadership Questionnaire* by Avolio, Gardner, and Walumbwa (2007) is available to use to a assess a preceptor's leadership authenticity. George, McLean, and Craig (2008) say leaders must model their own authenticity, passion, and leadership for their employees. Educators can facilitate experiences and provide knowledge to increase authenticity with the ultimate goal to improve preceptees' job satisfaction and retention.

Zilembo and Monterosso (2008) studied student nurses' perceptions of qualities that preceptors needed to be successful and found ($n = 22$) 96% of the students agreed preceptors should have strong leadership ability. The majority of students perceived the following characteristics as reflective of leadership and important for the preceptors to have: clinical competence, purposefulness, motivation, approachability, consistency, organization, and effective communication.

Transformational leaders are strongly associated with empowering nurses; a crucial attribute that will enable nurses to make innovative changes in their health care organization (Zilembo & Monterosso, 2008). As a result, mentors who empower their mentees will contribute to an overall mentoring culture in their work settings. Welch, past CEO of General Electric, has said in his book, *Winning* (2005), that at the end of the day it all comes down to winning for the employee and the employer. Although one might think of Jack Welch more as a manager and a highly respected CEO, he was also a leader that believed in permeating the workplace with a mentoring culture. He was not just geared to the organizational bottom line but insisted that employees feel satisfied and challenged, and not just accept the status quo.

Literature supports the notion that mentoring is viewed as an important developmental process that fosters professional maturation, career satisfaction, and the growth of strong, competent nurse leaders (Anthony et al., 2005; Shea & Gianotti, 2009; Stewart & Krueger, 1996). These authors also recognize that the closeness and cooperation that develops between a mentor and mentee over time produces great energy and creativity. It is this outpouring of ideas that assists the mentee and mentor to accomplish success. Shea and Gianotti (2009), Daloz (1999), Kram (1983), and Roberts (2000) agree that mentoring potential (or how a mentor or mentee will step up to the role of mentor or mentee) is an important predictor of what ultimately makes a good mentoring relationship. Think of some of the great mentor–mentee pairs: Socrates and Plato, Haydn and Beethoven, and Freud and Jung. It is the drawing out of the potential from the mentee and from the mentor that makes a huge difference.

Watkins (2003) shares effective strategies for leaders to use in transitioning to new work organizations that can be integrated into mentorships with new employees. He explains how to accelerate adjustment to new leadership positions with his $ST_ARS Model$ for recognizing portfolios, applauding individuals, identifying root causes of negative performance, and suggesting solutions. He emphasizes the importance of the first 90 days of a new work transition and suggests that this is when an employee needs support, and certainly some of this support could come from mentoring. Maxwell (2008) describes in his book, *Mentoring 101: What Every Leader Needs to Know,* how to assist leaders in developing effective mentorships for the individuals and their work organizations. Stoddard and Tamasy (2009) emphasize that leaders must provide a mentorship that sees the new employee as multidimensional and offer support, for the whole person and not just for the job performance.

Aiken (2005) and Kelly, McHugh, and Aiken (2011) conducted studies of professional practice at Magnet hospitals that are being linked with Kanter's (1979) investigation of workplace empowerment and demonstrate that healthy work environments allow for more nurse empowerment (Laschinger, Wilk, Cho, & Greco, 2009). This outcome has been identified as directly related to mentoring and effective leadership by nurses who practice in Magnet hospitals. Magnet status is known as the "gold standard" of nursing care quality (Abraham, Jerome-D'Emilia, & Begun, 2011). Of course it is not feasible to make sweeping generalizations that all nurses who work at Magnet hospitals perceive themselves as empowered or that they have received effective mentoring, but the majority appear to be empowered.

The American Association of Critical-Care Nurses (AACN) released *The AACN Standards for Establishing and Sustaining Healthy Work Environments: A Journey to Excellence* (2005a, 2005b). This document focuses on six areas that are mandatory if a safe and healthy work environment is to exist in hospitals: communication, collaboration, decision making, staffing, recognition, and leadership. The leaders need to come forward from the profession and take on responsibility for maintaining these standards. Nurses can and are stepping up to the plate in many settings and, perhaps with more coaching and mentoring, will join the crusade to establish a mentoring culture that will help produce a healthy work environment. More and more, it is the nurse manager and other nurse leaders who need to bring together the hospital executives and bedside nurses so that organizational and professional goals can be achieved. With the current demand for nurses, it is imperative that nurse leaders create positive work environments, socialize nurses to adapt new ways for delivering nursing care, and allow for development of leadership skills by all.

Educators can use a self-directed tool such as that developed by Riley-Doucet (2008) to assist staff nurses in being more prepared to precept nursing students. Likewise, *A Leadership & Management Competency Checklist* can be used as a guide in precepting nursing students and new graduates toward obtaining appropriate leadership and management experiences to accomplish their goals—similar to how nurses often use clinical skills checklists to orient new employees (Grossman, 2007).

Additionally, when there is great change and instability in a work environment there is decreased empowerment and job satisfaction (Kuokkanen, Suominen, Harkonen, Kukkurainen, & Doran, 2009). Nurse leaders can assist in helping nurses feel empowered, which will provide the momentum for nurses to want to stay in their positions and recruit and mentor more nurses. Also, new graduate nurses perceived a more effective precepting/mentoring experience when they had a preceptor who demonstrated caring behaviors and did not act like they were only precepting because their unit manager expected them to precept (Schumaker, 2007).

Whitmore (2009) describes how to "grow human potential" via coaching (a part of the mentorships for most mentees) for performance with his recommended principles of coaching and leadership. Gilley, Gilley, and Kouider (2010) suggest managerial coaching for improving employee performance. Basically, leaders need to be mentors and during the mentorships need to coach their mentees and possibly others' mentees regarding how to grow with the organization's work culture, how to contribute to making a mentoring culture, and how to pursue the organization's vision while at the same time accomplishing one's own career and personal goals. The importance of mentors introducing mentees to influential people who can help their careers may be the most significant outcome for the individual but will also positively impact the organization and profession. By creating a mentoring culture network, the profession can accomplish much more than if individuals work in isolation.

STRATEGIES TO MEASURE OUTCOMES OF MENTORING

Mentoring is positively correlated with salary growth, increased self-esteem, job and career satisfaction, and decreased turnover intentions for the mentee (Goran, 2001). All of these outcomes could easily be measured and positively influence the profession by improving the image of nursing. Hubbard (2010) recommends some easy-to-implement strategies for measuring outcomes in his book, *How to Measure Anything: Finding the Value of "Intangibles" in Business.* Bower (2000) describes that another important outcome of mentoring are the relationships that are generated. These tend to result in lasting and unique colleague contacts that could be tracked in longitudinal studies.

Mentoring experts validate that people who have worked successfully with a mentor have more promotions, increased incomes, increased career satisfaction, and increased mobility than those without mentors (Allen, Finkelstein, & Poteet, 2009; Dungy, 2010; Ensher & Murphy, 2005; Schwiebert, 2000; Zachary, 2005). The key to successful mentoring is collegiality and caring between the mentor, the mentee, and others in the organization (Kram, 1983). Perhaps a measurement of potential mentor caring would be helpful to determine if individuals would be a caring mentor and also, to suggest strategies for developing a more caring mentor. The *Caring Factor Survey* by Watson (2009) could be used as a measure of caring.

Kram (1983) believes that mentees (in academia and business) can advance even more if multiple mentors are involved with a mentee. For example, if a junior faculty in her first year of academia also practices one day/week in a primary care clinic, and additionally works in the Genetic Institute for 5 hours/week with a bench scientist, that individual will have a mentorship with a senior faculty who will assist with the academic aspect of teaching and try to connect her with people who can help her with her research trajectory. But also she will probably have some precepting every now and then regarding new policies and procedures at the clinic from the full-time APRNs, and will be coached on various laboratory procedures by the geneticist. She will also have some coaching on the details of her new position, her job description, and hopefully, politics of the department and university. This is an example of a multiple mentorship. It is common knowledge that the majority of faculty who have had mentors are more productive in obtaining competitive grants, leading professional organizations, and publishing more books and refereed journal articles. Kram also suggests that research is needed regarding the mentoring relationship in all stages of the mentorship and so she advocates the use of longitudinal studies (Kram, 1985).

Measuring mentoring, precepting, or coaching on collaborative learning units might be an effective method to collect outcome data since all disciplines assist with new employee orientation, and generally a collaborative leadership style and shared governance is in place on these multidisciplinary-friendly units (Budgen & Gamroth, 2008; Callaghan et al., 2009).

O'Keefe and Forrester (2009) studied the results of Magnet recognition at their institution and found that a successful online mentoring program between experienced and protégé RNs had the following outcomes:

1. Improved nurse satisfaction, recruitment, and retention
2. A change to a more positive perception of nurses by nurses at the institution and their co-workers
3. Increased support by nurses' co-workers
4. Improved patient care outcomes

The Magnet hospital movement began in 1980 and is based on the American Nurses Association's *Scope and Standards for Nurse Administrators* (2009). Magnet recognition is a process that assesses the implementation of five components of nursing excellence (American Nurses Credentialing Center [ANCC], 2012):

1. Transformational leadership
2. Structural empowerment
3. Exemplary professional practice
4. New knowledge, innovation, and improvement and
5. Empirical quality results

Mentorship programs are certainly vehicles that are used to arrive at the above mentioned excellence and are often described in the Magnet hospital literature. Aiken (2005) describes the results of a study that paired four Magnet hospitals in the United States with four hospitals in developing countries. Results indicated that nurses and hospital administrators have similar philosophies globally regarding the importance of quality improvement initiatives.

Magnet status, for excellence in nursing services, rewards workplaces that place a high premium on nursing services that empower and respect nursing staff. Magnet recognition fosters a collaborative practice and values contributions of nurses, educational support from nurses within the facility, the quality of patient care provided by the institution, research-based practices, shared governance structure that encourages nursing input on decisions regarding patient care, and promotion of an empowered nursing service. Magnet hospitals boast that their nurses are more satisfied with their jobs, which they say encourages nurses to perform at peak levels. Magnet status has also been shown to be a factor in attracting physicians of the highest caliber who want to work with a highly competent nursing staff. The Magnet Recognition Program sponsored by the ANCC is viewed by some as a catalyst for changing hospital environments. For example, one hospital wanted to focus on identifying qualities that have a positive long-term effect on nurses' job satisfaction and patient outcomes. The Magnet Recognition Program assisted this hospital in developing increased clinical autonomy, more opportunities for interdisciplinary relationships, and increased availability of resources. There are multiple accounts in the literature that share how specific institutions were able to gain Magnet accreditation (Jakubik, Ellades, Gavriloff, & Weese, 2011; Johnson, Billingsley, May, Costa, & Hanson, 2004; Taylor, 2005).

Another award given to hospitals reflects outcome excellence in critical care practice. It is the Beacon Award for Critical Care Excellence sponsored by the American Association of Critical-Care Nurses (AACN), which recognizes the highest-quality standards in nurse recruitment, retention, and patient outcomes in critical care services. (Applications, information questions, and requirements for obtaining recognition can be obtained in either the AACN News or online at www.aacn.org.)

EXAMPLES OF MEASURING MENTORING OUTCOMES

Suen and Chow (2001) developed a mentoring program adapted from the English National Board (ENB) for Nursing, Midwifery, and Health Visiting to use for program evaluation of mentorships in university nursing programs in Hong Kong. Using a framework comprising the five roles of a mentor as defined by the ENB (guide, counselor, friend, assistant, and adviser), they developed an evaluation questionnaire for mentee students to use in assessing the mentors. The tool consists of 33 questions. Demographics and two subjective questions requesting their perceptions of the mentoring experience were also completed by the mentees. Although no validity or reliability data on this tool were given, the tool could serve as a guide for obtaining other mentees' perceptions of their preceptors or mentors. Results from this study revealed several ways to improve mentor preparation for working more effectively with students.

Hayes (1998) found a positive relationship between mentoring and student self-efficacy in her study of 238 nurse practitioner students in their final semester. Hayes used *The Quality of Mentoring Tool* (Caine, 1989), a 14-item Likert-type scale that evaluates a person who was influential in the respondent's career development, the ways in which this was accomplished, and the significance of the relationship.

Reliability was reported at 0.95. Significant findings were generated. Nurse practitioner students who chose their own preceptor nurse practitioner had higher score on this instrument. The nurse practitioner students also identified the length of time they were assigned to the nurse practitioner and the preceptor's prior precepting experience. Interestingly, the areas that lowered the scores concerned indirect patient care activities or other nurse practitioner role functions such as research, consultation, case management, quality assurance, teaching, counseling, and influencing health policy. If the student had a physician assistant or physician as a preceptor, these scores were even lower. The variables that were the best predictors of mentor success were length of practicum time, with the longer the practicum the higher the mentoring score, and if the nurse practitioner preceptor had experience being a preceptor. Barker (2006), Szanton, Mihaly, Alhusen, and Becker (2010) and Harrington (2011) offer similar accounts of the advantages of mentoring and precepting in transitioning from the new graduate APRN to the competent APRN. The American Academy of Nurse Practitioners (2006) offer several documents to review on mentoring and mentorships on their website, accessible at www.aanp.org/AANPCMS2.

Cohen (1998a, 1999, 2000) offers self-assessment instruments with interpretation and implications for mentor–employee relationships. Cohen (1998b) has also developed a video and guides for mentors and mentees. No data regarding reliability and validity are offered regarding the tools.

Noe (1988) presents a tool to measure two scales assessing career (the extent to which the mentor provided exposure and visibility, sponsorship, protection, and challenging assignments) and psychosocial (the degree to which the mentor served as a role model and provided counseling, acceptance, and confirmation) functions of mentoring with a 29-item Likert-like response. Internal consistency reliability for the career-related scale was .89 and for the psychosocial functions scale was .92. The tool could be applicable to measuring mentees' perceptions of their mentor functions in nursing.

MENTORS AND MENTEES

Several have published their overwhelmingly positive experiences with working with preceptors, nurses, and student nurses. For example, Boswell and Wilhoit (2004) interviewed 67 new RNs regarding their perceptions of nurse practice quality. The nurses identified comprehensive orientation, continuing education, and mentoring as constituting high-quality practice. Papp, Markkanen, and von Bonsdorff (2003) cite findings from their study of 16 nursing students' perceptions of positive learning environments as including quality mentoring by staff nurses. Bernard (2004) describes positive outcomes regarding attitudes on aging and working with the terminally ill after students had specific role modeling with these patient populations. Certainly, shadowing a role model can generate positive learning for mentees who have identified specific types of activities they are interested in observing. Mentees who are assigned a mentor or preceptor without delineating a specific purpose for the experience will likely not achieve their goals. Dunn, Ehrich, Mylonas, and Hansford (2000) conducted a phenomenological study of 25 teachers and 14 nurse students in their final semester field experience of their baccalaureate program who had been assigned a preceptor. The purpose of the research was to determine the participants' perceptions of the experience and the outcomes generated from the preceptorship, which included:

- *Role integration.* Students felt they were deemed competent by a contributing member of the organization, their preceptor.
- *Increased confidence.* Students confirmed their self-efficacy and refocused their commitment to the profession due to their improved self-concept after working with a mentor.
- *Altruism.* Students felt they made a difference in their patients' or learners' lives.

Students shared multiple interactions they had been a part of with their mentors as the "most influential" aspect of the preceptorship.

Pinkerton (2003) described an 18-month mentoring program used in her institution to increase retention of RNs. Mentors cited that they felt empowered and related a higher job satisfaction after having experienced mentoring a new nurse. Mentees felt they gained increased self-confidence, optimism about the future, and increased critical thinking skills. This program was responsible for a 3% decrease in turnover in its first 18 months of inception. Myrick (2002) also found that "preceptors were more likely to assist with fostering critical thinking indirectly through their role modeling, facilitating, guiding, and prioritizing than they were to directly impact preceptees' critical thinking ability through questioning" (p. 161). This finding is significant because it validates the importance of having new nurses and students experience shadowing or observing proficient or expert nurses during their orientation. Experiential learning or working with a preceptor or mentor in everyday practice can assist students in appreciating how theory and research findings direct practice. This is a significant outcome of precepting and mentoring. Using Bandura's (1977) Social Learning Theory as a conceptual framework justifies the use of shadowing or observational experiences with expert nurses as yielding strong learning outcomes. Nursing students learn by watching procedures performed by staff, peers, and instructors, which leads to vicarious learning. Modeling is another method of professional socialization. According to Bandura there are two criteria for successful modeling: (1) the role model must be competent, and (2) there must be opportunities for students to practice. Then the mentee has a conscious purpose to model himself or herself after the mentor. Luhanga, Billay, Grundy, Myrick, and Yonge (2010) describe how valuable the one-on-one preceptor–preceptee relationship is for gaining professional knowledge, skills, and values—much more so than simulation and college laboratory experiences. Additionally, working one-on-one with an experienced RN can assist with socializing the new nurse into the profession.

One hospital implemented a mentoring program for their Labor & Delivery Unit and Newborn Intensive Care Unit after finding a 20% turnover rate of new graduate RNs in 1 year. After the mentoring program the turnover rate dropped to 7% in 1 year. This increase in retention of RNs saved the hospital $328,800 and was attributed to the mentoring program (Faron & Poeltler, 2007). Partnerships between hospitals and colleges of nursing have also documented annual savings due to mentoring between faculty, staff, and students as a result of their partnerships (Novotny, Donahue, & Bhalla, 2004). Cost savings documented included less expenditure on recruitment ($79,500), employing travel nurses ($48,750), and employing adjunct faculty ($30,688). Tracy, Jagsi, Starr, and Tarbell (2003) studied the outcomes of a faculty mentoring program and found that having a role model, having increased visibility, and having someone to turn to if needed were perceived as invaluable for success by junior faculty.

It is well established that many nurses burn out and leave the profession. Raiger (2005) presents a review of the literature on burnout in nursing that offers data to support the need for mutual trust and support, vertical communication channels, and recognition of nurses. This seems to be analogous to what a mentoring culture would provide. Findings indicate that fostering trust, open communication, and respect protects nurses from burnout and facilitates a healthy work environment. More mentors need to intervene in the health care settings and transform work settings for nurses. Almada, Carafoli, Flattery, French, and McNamera (2004) and Reeves (2004) suggest several ideas that have assisted their institutions in retaining nurses by using a mentoring program. Greene and Puetzer (2002) used clinical tracking forms, planning calendars, and feedback mechanisms to increase their communication between mentors and mentees regarding skill and knowledge development for new nurses. Having a mentoring program helped increase retention and recruitment, as well as reinforced the need to build relationships between experienced and new nurses. Greggs-McQuilkin (2004) suggests that nursing assures a mentoring mentality. She says that the profession needs to mentor for survival since it is the interrelationships with one another that will be key to successful goal achievement for nursing. She advises nurses to focus more on collaborating and less on competing in their work settings in order to create environments in which respect, sharing, learning, and support are the standard instead of the unusual.

CONCLUSION

After reviewing the literature, few data based articles were located that delineated outcomes of mentoring. All pointed to the need for continuing relationships between new and experienced staff, which is specifically what mentoring models such as reverse, multiple, and co-mentoring will foster. Noe, Greenberger, and Wang (2002) suggested several strategies for future mentoring models and recommended more measurement of outcomes. For example, measurements of mentees' salary growth over their careers, promotion rates at various institutions, and number of mentees mentored in the future would be helpful. A longitudinal study that spanned 20 or 30 years of careers of nurses who had been mentored versus nurses without mentoring would be useful. Maintaining connections with all nurses will assist in expanding the mentoring culture in nursing. As Kaplan and Norton (2004) advocate, "There is no asset with greater potential for an organization than the collective knowledge possessed by all of its employees" (p. 63). Sometimes the most significant outcomes are intangible and cannot be measured with benchmark indicators. Collegiality between employees in one's healthy work setting may well be the ultimate outcome of a mentoring culture that will facilitate more teamwork and eventual vital productivity.

REFERENCES

Abraham, J., Jerome-D'Emilia, B., & Begun, J. (2011). The diffusion of magnet hospital recognition. *Health Care Management Review, 36*(4), 306–314.

Aiken, L. H. (2005). Journey to excellence. *Reflection on Nursing Leadership, 1,* 16–19.

Allen, T. D., & Eby, L. T. (2004). Factors related to mentor reports of mentoring functions provided: Gender and relational characteristics. *Sex Roles, 50*(1–2), 129–139.

Allen, T. D., Eby, L. T., O'Brien, K. E., & Lentz, E. (2008). The state of mentoring research: A qualitative review of current research methods and future research implications. *Journal of Vocational Behavior, 73,* 343–357.

Allen, T. D., Finkelstein, L., & Poteet, M. L. (2009). *Designing workplace mentoring programs: An evidence based approach.* Malden, MA: Blackwell Publishing.

Almada, P., Carafoli, K., Flattery, J., French, D., & McNamera, M. (2004). Improving the retention rate of newly graduated nurses. *Journal for Nurses in Staff Development, 20,* 268–273.

American Academy of Nurse Practitioners. (2006). *Mentoring assessment.* Retrieved from http://www.aanp.org/AANPCMS2

American Association of Critical-Care Nurses. (2005a). *The AACN Standards for establishing and sustaining healthy work environments: A journey to excellence.* Retrieved from http://www.aacn.org/wd/hwe/content/hwehome .pcms?menu=hwe

American Association of Critical-Care Nurses. (2005b). Healthy work environments. *AACN News, 22,* 2.

American Nurses Association. (2009). *Scope and standards for nurse administrators.* Washington, DC: Author.

American Nurses Credentialing Center. (2012). *American nurses credentialing center magnet recognition.* Retrieved from http://www.nursecredentialing .org/Magnet.aspx

Anthony, M., Standing, T., Glick, J., Duffy, M., Paschall, F., Sauer, M.,... Dumpe, M. L. (2005). Leadership and nurse retention: The pivotal role of nurse managers. *Journal of Nursing Administration, 35,* 146–155.

Avolio, B. J., Gardner, W. L., Walumbwa, F. O., Luthans, F., & May, D. R. (2004). Unlocking the mask: A look at the process by which authentic leaders impact follower attitudes and behaviors. *Leadership Quarterly, 15,* 801–823.

Avolio, B. J., Gardner, W. L., & Walumbwa, F. O. (2007). *Authentic leadership questionnaire* [web document]. Retrieved from http://www.mindgarden .com/products/alq.htm

Bandura, A. (1977). *Social learning theory.* Englewood Cliffs, NJ: Prentice Hall.

Barker, E. R. (2006). Mentoring: A complex relationship. *Journal of the American Academy of Nurse Practitioners, 18,* 56–61.

Beecroft, P. C., Dorey, F., & Wenten, M. (2008). Turnover intention in new graduate nurses: A multivariate analysis. *Journal of Advanced Nursing, 62,* 41–52.

Benner, P. (1984). *From novice to expert: Excellence and power in clinical nursing practice.* Menlo Park, CA: Addison-Wesley.

Bernard, M. (2004). Overcoming ageism, one student at a time: Mentoring programs improve student attitudes toward older patients. *Geriatrics, 59,* 11.

Boswell, S., & Wilhoit, K. (2004). New nurses' perceptions of nursing practice and quality patient care. *Journal of Nursing Care Quality, 19,* 76–81.

Bower, F. (2000). *Nurses taking the lead: Personal qualities of effective leadership.* Philadelphia, PA: W. B. Saunders.

Budgen, C., & Gamroth, L. (2008). An overview of practice education models. *Nurse Education Today, 28,* 273–283.

Caine, R. (1989). Mentoring the novice clinical nurse specialist. *Clinical Nurse Specialist, 3,* 76–78.

Callaghan, D., Watts, W., McCullough, D., Moreau, J., Little, M., Gamroth, L., & Durnford, K. (2009). The experience of two practice education models: Collaborative learning unit and preceptorship. *Nurse Education in Practice, 9,* 244–252.

Cary, S. (2008). Mentoring generations today for tomorrow's leaders. *Nephrology Nursing Journal, 35*(2), 118–119.

Cohen, N. (1998a). *The principles of adult mentoring inventory.* Amherst, MA: HRD Press.

Cohen, N. (1998b). *The mentor critique form.* Amherst, MA: HRD Press.

Cohen, N. (2000). *Becoming a mentor: A video based workshop.* Amherst, MA: HRD Press.

Daloz, L. (1999). *Mentor: Guiding the journey of adult learners* (2nd ed.). San Francisco, CA: Jossey-Bass.

Dungy, T. (2010). *The mentor leader: Secrets to building people and teams that win consistently.* Carol Stream, IL: Tyndale House Publishers.

Dunn, S., Ehrich, L., Mylonas, A., & Hansford, B. (2000). Students' perceptions of field experience in professional development: A comparative study. *Journal of Nursing Education, 39,* 393–400.

Ensher, E. A., & Murphy, S. (2005). *Power mentoring: How successful mentors and protégés get the most out of their relationships.* San Francisco, CA: Jossey-Bass.

Erikson, E. (1963). *Childhood and society* (2nd ed.). NY: Norton.

Faron, S., & Poeltler, D. (2007). Growing our own, inspiring growth and increasing retention through mentoring. *Nursing in Women's Health, 11*(2), 139–143.

George, B., McLean, A., & Craig, N. (2008). *Finding your true north – A personal guide.* San Francisco, CA: Jossey-Bass.

Giallonardo, L. M., Wong, C. A., & Iwasiw, C. L. (2010). Authentic leadership of preceptors: Predictor of new graduate nurses' work engagement and job satisfaction. *Journal of Nursing Management, 18,* 993–1003.

Gilley, A., Gilley, J., & Kouider, E. (2010). Characteristics of managerial coaching. *Performance Improvement Quarterly, 23*(1), 53–70.

Goran, S. (2001). Mentorship as a teaching strategy. *Critical Care Nursing Clinics of North America, 13,* 119–129.

Greene, M., & Puetzer, M. (2002). The value of mentoring: A strategic approach to retention and recruitment. *Journal of Nursing Care Quality, 17,* 63–70.

Greggs-McQuilkin, D. (2004). Mentoring really matters: Motivate and mentor a colleague. *MEDSURG Nursing, 13,* 209, 266.

Grossman, S. (2007) Assisting critical care nurses in acquiring leadership skills: Development of a leadership & management competency checklist. *Dimensions of Critical Care Nursing, 26*(2), 57–65.

Harrington, S. (2011). Mentoring new nurse practitioners to accelerate their development as primary care providers: A literature review. *Journal of American Academy of Nurse Practitioners, 23*(4), 168–174.

Hayes, E. (1998). Mentoring and nurse practitioner student self-efficacy. *Western Journal of Nursing Research, 20,* 521–535.

Hubbard, D. (2010). *How to measure anything: Finding the value of "intangibles" in business.* Hoboken, NJ: John Wiley & Sons.

Institute of Medicine. (2010). *The future of nursing: Leading change, advancing health.* Washington, DC: National Academies Press.

Jakubik, L. D., Ellades, A. B., Gavriloff, C. L., & Weese, M. M. (2011). Nurse mentoring study demonstrates a magnetic work environment: Predictors of mentoring benefits among pediatric nurses. *Journal of Pediatric Nursing, 26*(2), 156–164.

Johnson, J., Billingsley, M., May, C., Costa, L., & Hanson, K. (2004). Cause célèbre: Georgetown University Hospital's journey to magnet. *Policy, Politics, and Nursing Practice, 5,* 217–227.

Kanter, R. (1979). Power failure in management circuits. *Harvard Business Review, 57,* 65–75.

Kaplan, R., & Norton, D. (2004). Measuring the strategic readiness of intangible assets. *Harvard Business Review, 82,* 52–63, 121.

Kelly, L. S., McHugh, M. D., & Aiken, L. H. (2011). Nurse outcomes in magnet and non-magnet hospitals. *Journal of Nursing Administration, 41*(10), 428–433.

Kram, K. (1983). Phases of the mentor relationship. *Academy of Management Journal, 26,* 608–625.

Kram, K. (1985). *Mentoring at work: Developmental relationships in organizational life.* Glenview, IL: Scott Foresman.

Kuokkanen, L., Suominen, T., Harkonen, E., Kukkurainen, M. L., & Doran, D. (2009). Effects of organizational change on work-related empowerment, employee satisfaction, and motivation. *Nursing Administration Quarterly, 33*(2), 116–124.

Laschinger, H. K., Wilk, R., Cho, J., & Greco, P. (2009). Empowerment, engagement and perceived effectiveness in nursing work environments: Does experience matter? *Journal of Nursing Management, 17,* 636–646.

Levinson, D., Darrow, C., Klein, E., Levinson, M., & McKee, B. (1978). *The seasons of a man's life.* New York, NY: Knopf.

Luhanga, F. L., Billay, D., Grundy, Q., Myrick, F., & Yonge, O. (2010). The one-to-one relationship: Is it really key to an effective preceptorship experience? A review of the literature. *International Journal of Nursing Education Scholarship, 7*(1), Article 21, 1–15.

Luna, G., & Cullen, D. (2000). *Empowering the faculty: Mentoring redirected and renewed.* Washington, DC: George Washington University Press.

Maxwell, J. C. (2008). *Mentoring 101: What every leader needs to know.* Nashville, TN: Thomas Nelson.

Myrick, F. (2002). Preceptorship and critical thinking in nursing education. *Journal of Nursing Education, 41,* 154–164.

Nedd, N., Nash, M., Galindo-Ciocon, D., & Belgrave, G. (2006). Guided growth intervention from novice to expert through a mentoring program. *Journal of Nursing Care Quality, 21*(1), 20–23.

Noe, R. (1988). An investigation of the determinants of successful assigned mentoring relationships. *Personnel Psychology, 41,* 457–479.

Noe, R., Greenberger, B., & Wang, S. (2002). Mentoring: What we know and where we might go. *Research in Personnel and Human Resource Management, 21,* 124–173.

Novotny, J., Donahue, M., & Bhalla, B. (2004). The clinical partnership as strategic alliance. *Journal of Professional Nursing, 20,* 216–221.

O'Keefe, T., & Forrester, D. A. (2009). A successful online mentoring program for nurses. *Nursing Administration Quarterly, 33*(3), 245–250.

Papp, I., Markkanen, M., & von Bonsdorff, M. (2003). Clinical environment as a learning environment: Student nurses' perceptions concerning clinical learning experiences. *Nurse Education Today, 23,* 262–268.

Pinkerton, S. (2003). Mentoring new graduates. *Nursing Economics, 21,* 202–203.

Raiger, J. (2005). Applying a cultural lens to the concept of burnout. *Journal of Transcultural Nursing, 16,* 71–76.

Reeves, K. (2004). Nurses nurturing nurses: A mentoring program. *Nurse Leader, 2,* 47–49, 53.

Riley-Doucet, C. (2008). A self-directed learning tool for nurses who precept student nurses. *Journal for Nurses in Staff Development, 24,* E7–E14.

Roberts, A. (2000). Mentoring revisited: A phenomenological reading of the literature. *Mentoring and Tutoring, 8,* 145–170.

Schwiebert, V. (2000). *Mentoring: Creating connected, empowered relationships,* Alexandria, VA: American Counseling Association.

Schumaker, D. L. (2007). Caring behaviors or preceptors and perceived by new graduate orientees. *Journal for Nurses in Staff Development, 23,* 186–192.

Shea, G. F., & Gianotti, S. C. (2009). *Mentoring: Make it a mutually rewarding experience.* Menlo Park, CA: Crisp Learning.

Stewart, B., & Krueger, L. (1996). An evolutionary concept analysis of mentoring in nursing. *Journal of Professional Nursing, 12,* 311–321.

Stoddard, D. A., & Tamasy, R. J. (2009). *The heart of mentoring: Ten proven principles.* Colorado Springs, CO: NAVPRESS.

Suen, L., & Chow, F. (2001). Students' perceptions of the effectiveness of mentors in an undergraduate nursing program in Hong Kong. *Journal of Advanced Nursing, 36,* 505–511.

Szanton, S. L., Mihaly, L. K., Alhusen, J., & Becker, K. L. (2010). Taking charge of the challenge: Factors to consider in taking your first nurse practitioner job. *Journal of the American Academy of Nursing, 22,* 356–360.

Taylor, N. (2005). The magnet pull. *Nursing Management, 36,* 36–41.

Tracy, E., Jagsi, R., Starr, R., & Tarbell, N. (2003). Outcomes of a pilot faculty mentoring program. *American Journal of Obstetrics and Gynecology, 191,* 1846–1850.

Wagner, A. L. (2008). Caring mentorship. *International Journal for Human Caring, 12*(2), 95.

Watkins, M. (2003). *The first ninety days: Critical success strategies for new leaders at all levels.* Boston, MA: Harvard Business School Press.

Watson, J. (2009). *Assessment and measuring caring in nursing and health science.* (2nd ed.). New York, NY: Springer.

Welch, J. (2005). *Winning.* New York, NY: Harper Collins.

Whitmore, J. (2009). *Coaching for performance – Growing human potential and purpose: The principles and practices of coaching and leadership* (4th ed.). Boston, MA: Nicholas Brealey Publishing.

Zachary, L. (2005). *Creating a mentoring culture: The organization's guide.* San Francisco, CA: Jossey-Bass.

Zilembo, M., & Monterosso, L. (2008). Nursing students' perceptions of desirable leadership qualities in nurse preceptors: A descriptive survey. *Contemporary Nurse, 27,* 194–206.

8

Building a Mentoring Culture in Nursing: Implications for the Future

ENCOURAGING TO MENTOR OTHERS

Mentoring is not something to take lightly, and although one purpose of this book is to stimulate more nurses to become part of the mentoring culture, not everyone may be able, or may not want, to be a successful nurse mentor. They can, however, be effective at an aspect of mentoring. Just as leaders are made and not born (Bennis, 2003), nurses can be taught the skills of mentoring or they can acquire them by being mentored by an effective mentor. They cannot be taught the art of encouraging others, however. Someone who is not self-empowered and self-confident cannot encourage or lead others to become empowered. More than likely, her or his work setting is not conducive for encouraging others and working collaboratively. If it is a clinical setting, it is probably an extremely task-oriented and unfriendly atmosphere under the leadership of an enabling manager, or, if it is an academic setting, it is most likely a competitive, cutthroat, or uncaring environment.

Advancing a mentoring culture is necessary and timely for the profession as well as for every nurse—who can help to develop this professional network by beginning early. Due to our chaotic health care system and volatile economy, there has never been a greater need for nurses to gain new skills and knowledge to empower themselves. Moreover, many health care institutions are expanding into vast conglomerates with multiple health care systems, some of which may not employ nurses or are transferring nursing positions to less educated and less costly employees. One reason why nurses must be involved in any assessments for change, new planning, and decision making in health care is to ensure that nurses play a part, and lead in, every microsystem that any health care organization newly establishes or sustains. For their part, senior leaders involved in planning should be connected to people with authority and possess the negotiating skills to gain or keep what is best for nursing. With innovative ideas for creating more effective care delivery, the escalating growth in technology, and the burgeoning costs of health care, it is not difficult to realize that care delivery cannot continue as it has. Having a flourishing mentoring culture in nursing will assist the profession to grow exponentially and, at the same time, create strong bonds between nurses, which will assist in protecting nursing jobs and the profession. This chapter discusses ways to encourage mentoring, advantages of early networking for building careers and the profession, creative incentives for the mentor and mentee, and the influence of a mentoring culture within nursing, health care work organizations, and the overall mentor and mentee relationship.

Advantages of Early Networking for Building Careers and the Profession

Chitty and Black (2011) say that "mentoring" is often the answer when successful nurses are asked: "What has been most helpful to you in your becoming a successful clinician, educator, or researcher?" One may wonder, "How come I did not get connected to someone who could help me with my career when I was in school?" Here are the questions that people who feel entitled, *not* empowered, keep asking themselves: "How come I am still doing the same thing and getting nowhere fast?" and "Where was the mentoring connection for me?"

If graduate school was not part of a nurse's career path, he or she may have missed out on the most frequent context for connecting to mentors. Still, there are other possibilities, including connecting with others in professional organizations, colleagues at work, or college friends. What about keeping in touch with one of your professors from school? What about considering graduate school now? How about talking with the clinical instructor who teaches nursing students on the unit? Why not seek collaboration with some of the affiliating colleges of nursing? Perhaps there is an opportunity to get involved with teaching in the college skills laboratory, tutoring students, or making a presentation at your state nursing organization that will lead to becoming part of a mentoring network.

Not only is early networking in one's profession important but so is making connections informally and formally with individuals we encounter every day. Daniel Goleman echoes this sentiment in his 1999 edition of *Working with Emotional Intelligence,* where he says: "The rules for work are changing. We're being judged by a new yardstick: not just by how smart we are, or by our training and expertise, but also by how well we handle ourselves and each other"(p. 3).

In today's workforce, this is even truer. For example, Donna and Claire started as new graduates from the same BSN program on a high acuity medical unit in a teaching hospital about 10 years ago. When Donna was asked to help with the student nurses or precept a new employee, she always put it in terms of self-interest, of what she got from it? "No," she'd respond, "I am unable to come to a staff barbecue at the unit manager's house unless I get paid; No, I cannot change my weekend off since another staff member has a wedding;" and the list goes on. Donna left the institution after about 16 months and found a position on a similar high acuity medical unit at a nearby hospital. For her part, Claire volunteered to help the students when they were on the unit; agreed to precept new staff and even developed a new checklist for clinical skill competency evaluation; always attended out-of-work events such as the unit manager's barbecue; and was flexible with schedule changes whenever she possibly could. Claire also joined the Multidisciplinary AIDS Research Team as a new graduate and continues to work voluntarily with the project. Today Donna, Clinical Level I nurse, is working three 12-hour night shifts at a neighboring hospital and is always complaining about the institution, the unit, the staff and the patients she works with on the unit. Claire has obtained a master's degree as a Family Nurse Practitioner (FNP) and works full time as a FNP in the hospital's Primary Care Clinic, and also does clinical teaching for a group of senior nursing students on eight Saturdays/ year on her previous unit. She maintains her per diem RN status on the unit and has continued to work with the Multidisciplinary AIDS Research Team. She is happy with her FNP position and is co-planning the 10-year alumni celebration for her graduating class. Her work with the AIDS Research Team has been published in five different venues and she is frequently asked to present on her aspect of the AIDS project. She has also been selected for a fellowship to begin her doctorate in nursing at the university.

What is it that made Donna leave her first hospital and Claire stay on? The literature has focused on trying to increase retention rates of new graduates and nurses in general but, often times, to no avail. Mitchell, Holton, Lee, Sablynski, and Erez (2001), for example, recommended that human resource departments examine what it was that retained certain employees instead of focusing on the factors that propelled staff to leave. A new term, *job embeddedness,* was coined and Halfer and Graf (2006), Halfer (2007), Halfer, Graf, and Sullivan (2008), and Halfer (2011) studied this phenomenon with nurses. Halfer and Graf developed a tool, the Job/Work Environment Satisfaction Survey, and measured new graduates' perceptions of competence, professional development, practice support, work schedules, becoming part of a team, resource accessibility, and professional respect, and from this information developed a comprehensive internship program. In 2008, they used a longitudinal data collection design and measured pediatric nurses' perceptions with this tool. They also found a significantly decreased rate—from 20% to a 12% loss—in number of graduate nurses that left who previously experienced an internship. In terms of retaining new graduates, Park and Jones (2010) also found that, at the 3-year mark, when many new nurses leave the hospital, there were three variables that seemed to influence employees:

1. Fit of the job with other aspects of their life
2. Links with other employees
3. Level of sacrifice employees were willing to make in giving up these relationships or links with the other employees

It thus seems that an ongoing mentoring culture provides a strong link among employees that is difficult to give up. Also, it has been found that retention rates improve with a mentoring culture. Health care organizations can also work to strengthen employee links by offering child care facilities, gyms, libraries, or retail shops that are within close proximity to the hospital or are in the hospital and perhaps at a discount to hospital employees.

It is crucial to start networking early, otherwise we will not accomplish our goals. If we wait, it will get tougher and tougher to network and become part of *the* group that comprises the network. And the easiest way to network is to be introduced and connected by our mentors and our mentees.

Regarding connecting with people via informal versus formal lines in the organization and/or the profession, Katzenbach and Khan (2010) recommend using both the formal approach, which consists of strategy, structures, processes and procedures, programs, initiatives, performance goals, and metrics, along with all of the informal elements of an organization's communication system. Or, as they call it: "magic of the informal," which includes shared values, informal networks, communities, and pride. They also say that informal networks are generally fueled by peers and not the upper echelon of the organization. In fact, the upper management may be unaware of these networks. This would be a *huge* mistake for a nurse leader or manager to not be aware of the networks. These informal and formal networks are also necessary to enrich leadership succession planning for health care organizations and schools of nursing (Ponti, 2009).

Creative Incentives for Mentors and Mentees

First things first regarding the benefits for mentors: One needs to provide them with adequate training and preparation to be an effective mentor. Likewise, mentors need to have the resources to appropriately mentor the mentees (Jokelinen, Turunen, Tossavainen, Jamookeeah, & Coco; 2011). Another area that mentors and mentees are interested in are the possible measurable benefits that they experience through the relationship. Jakubik (2008) developed a tool for precisely this purpose, the *Jakubik Mentoring Benefits Questionnaire*, which can be used to measure mentorship benefits. In fact, Jakubik, Ellades, and Gavriloff (2012), who used the Jakubik Tool to predict mentoring benefits among pediatric nurses, found one benefit quite clearly—the evolution of a healthy work environment.

Another benefit for both the mentors and mentees is that they will become re-empowered or empowered, which will strengthen them and encourage them to pursue their goals (Gilmore, Kopeikin, & Douche, 2007). Mentors and mentees also greatly benefit from their mentorship(s) because they have a built-in sounding board to discuss new ideas. Most of the time mentees will give as much to the mentor as the mentee receives from the mentor or, in some instances, even more. Think of the technological savvy an experienced mentor can learn from a mentee who has recently graduated from his or her program as well as new ways to think about topics that are mutually interesting to both the mentor and mentee. Some mentors gain a keen understanding of their own children after working with a mentee who also most probably is a member of the mentor's children's generation.

Meister and Willyerd (2010) detail some pragmatic strategies and tools that can assist mentors in attracting the best workers or mentees and also help them in mentoring them to do their best work. Additionally, if mentors were to review Kiefer and Schlesinger's (2010) book, *Action Trumps Everything: Creating What You Want in an Uncertain World*, they would benefit by improving their entrepreneurial skills and also improving their abilities to make crucial decisions regarding the workplace. There are multiple benefits for the mentor and mentee that have already been discussed in previous chapters, but one of the most significant benefits for a mentee would be an opportunity "to achieve a new direction in his or her life" (p. 167) from shadowing a mentor/role model/coach (Metcalfe, 2010).

IMPACT OF HAVING A MENTORING CULTURE FOR THE NURSING PROFESSION

Just about every nursing professional organization newsletter or journal cites how critical it is for nurses to mentor others. And most organizations have a process by which members can network and obtain mentoring or coaching. Today, when health care is constantly changing and new roles such as anesthesiologist assistant (candidates for this program must have a BS or BA and then do 2 years in this program) are developing, there is more need to mentor and protect the scope of the role of nurse anesthetists and nurse practitioners as well as our registered nurses.

Once again, the concept of mentoring may be used too freely, and some may feel what an organization is really sponsoring is a year of coaching, not mentoring. It will depend on the mentor and mentee as to just what transpires. However, coaching a mentee to conduct research, present findings, and publish in a refereed journal; or develop an evidence-based practice protocol and disseminate its use; or apply for funding for a project is assisting someone to increase his or her leadership skills and is a viable way of providing mentorship.

Some nurses are caring for their families and parents, are very involved with their children's school organizations, or have multiple other responsibilities that do not allow time for anything else in their day. This is where a new way of thinking needs to begin that will allow the staff nurse a specific amount of time at work each shift to work on a topic, an intervention, a patient case, or some area that interests the nurse to research. (Of course, sometimes this time may not be available depending on the staffing and patient acuity.) Moreover, there will need to be more delegation, more use of a team care approach, and a generally different way of thinking that every task needs the nurse involved. From this initial work, it will be possible to develop ideas to explore further the specific topic a nurse is interested in researching. The nurse will develop a better understanding of this topic and can share with others at work, through a satellite outpatient program of the health care affiliation, at a college of nursing, on a website, or in a journal article. The nurse will begin to make connections with other people interested in similar topics. Zachary (2005) provides a *Mentoring Culture Audit* (consisting of 50 items) that will assist your unit or organization in developing a mentoring culture that best fits your needs. The tool is divided into two parts: I. Building Blocks consisting of Connecting Culture & Mentoring, and Infrastructure; and II. Hallmarks including Alignment, Accountability, Communication, Value & Visibility, Demand, Multiple Mentoring Opportunities, Education & Training, and Safety Nets (p. 272).

The nurse has now entered the mentoring culture and can decide how much time and effort to spend in maximizing the growth of his or her project. The nurse can study everything available on the topic and implement some evidence-based practice interventions that no one else has yet documented. Perhaps the nurse will begin to do some consulting work. Or maybe the nurse will decide to change career paths. Whatever choices are made, the nurse has the power to make a difference with this expertise. Most likely the nurse will find, as Chitty and Black (2011) stated, that along the road to new success, he or she was given advice and guided by others and thereby connected with the mentoring culture. The nurse will become passionate about the chosen work and learn all that he or she can on the subject, but eventually will probably want to use the findings to make a difference. By making a difference, the nurse will most likely be empowered to make some other changes regarding his or her work. By role modeling to other nurses that things do not have to revolve around task lists at the bedside or doing all of the paperwork developed for every patient, the nurse can inspire and encourage other nurses to change too. Some of the current work done by RNs needs to be redistributed to the team. Patients and families can also participate on the team. In many instances, the nurse can assist the patient to empower himself or herself to change habits and try new ways of promoting health. Registered nurses can gain recognition for their new ways of leading in patient care and in this way benefit the entire nursing profession.

Today, every nurse needs to be involved in a mentor network. It is now possible for more people than ever before to work together with more people on more projects from different corners of the Earth and on a more equal footing. In fact, Zachary (2009) says the most significant reasons for an organization to become successful is 1. having effective relationships, and 2. assisting workers in learning. How better to accomplish these two parameters than by establishing a mentoring culture? She calls this process group mentoring (which is similar to multiple mentoring except everyone is involved) and suggests three different ways to initiate it at a workplace: 1. Facilitated group mentoring, 2. Peer-group mentoring, or 3. Team group mentoring. Katzenbach and Khan (2010) have a good example of a tool to measure your organization's readiness for a change.

Work is being outsourced to areas in the world where skilled individuals will do the job effectively and more efficiently than if the work remained in the United States. Even radiographs are being sent out for interpretation in India, since it is considered more cost-effective to do so. These changes in health care delivery are being made every day, and most individuals are unaware. "So what?" one might ask. That is the key question because the answer is not clear. It would behoove the nursing profession to develop more connections with other disciplines and keep abreast of new technology and determine how it affects nursing care. Nurses need to visualize their work more broadly and create answers for the "So what?" questions. Keeping connected will help. Chief executive officers (CEOs), lawyers, accountants, entrepreneurs, and physicians can all network with nurses to expand networks.

Today, there are multiple settings for nurses to make a difference. Whether it is being involved in multidisciplinary projects, new trials of interventions, out-of-hospital health promotion activities, public health initiatives, media, journalism, or legislative work, there is a need for nursing input. Nurses need leadership skills as well as clinical skills to perform their work. The strongest mentoring appears to be occurring in academia, with nursing doctoral students and new faculty employed at research institutions. Outcome studies are necessary to validate that obtaining federal funding, promotion and tenure, and overall career success are directly correlated with the use of mentoring structures found in some academic settings. Success with strengthening the science of nursing is directly related to the productivity of these nurse scientists. However, having a mentoring culture that involves the majority of nurses—those who practice and work with patients on a regular basis—will be most advantageous for the profession since every nurse can add to the state of the science with findings from his or her everyday practice.

IMPACT OF HAVING A MENTORING CULTURE
FOR WORK ORGANIZATIONS

Satterly (2003) writes that many staff nurses feel overwhelmed and unsafe in their clinical settings and are moving out of the acute care arena to other health care facilities or even out of nursing all together. Her book, *Where Have All the Nurses Gone?*, explains how nurses are under siege and stressed with the declining quality of care that is generally being given in the United States. Many nurses at the bedside feel they are operating without enough support from their administrations.

Problems include not enough professional staff, poorly prepared nurses to care for higher-acuity patients, not enough properly trained ancillary workers, and lack of resources for implementing best practice care. Organizations have learned that in order to retain experienced nurses and recruit new nurses, well-developed, planned preceptorships are mandatory. Accounts in the literature describe partnering preceptorships and mentorships with Schools of Nursing even before the new graduate is hired in some areas of the country. Multiple articles detail the organization's gain in retention of nurses, lower nurse attrition rates, and improved morale when good precepting and mentoring are offered.

Chapter 4 in this book details how to set up mentorships and preceptorships in health care agencies, mentoring relationships in academia, and other supportive mentoring models for graduate and undergraduate education. Organizations are developing more supportive programs for nurses with specialty training, advanced programs for specialty units, and day-long workshops for nurses in a variety of areas such as legal, ethical, caring for the dying, documentation, new technology, and a myriad of other interventions. Some institutions are offering leadership workshops as well. Heifetz, Grashow, and Linsky (2009) suggest that the traditional theories of leadership are not capable of success in 2012, where constant chaos presents as such in most health care organizations. They recommend that leaders and mentors use never-been-thought-of-before communication methods and ways of relating to people in order to make a difference. They also offer some helpful points regarding what they have experienced when trying to inspire people that may be helpful to mentors. Conflict management and negotiation strategy workshops are helpful skills for all nurse leaders. Mentoring will enhance mentees' knowledge of the health care system, increase their confidence and scope of thinking, and develop their communication and collaboration skills.

With more partnerships forming between academia and clinical settings, more educational programs are planned for staff. For example, nurses in the community including nurse practitioners and the emergency department could use advice on how other hospitals have developed emergency preparedness protocols. This knowledge base has become essential for all nursing programs (Spain, Clements, DeRanieri, & Holt, 2012). Collaboration with nursing staff from various health care agencies, professional organizations, and other disciplines will help to develop excellent educational programs. Faculty and staff can collaborate on developing programs and sharing resources with staff and students.

Organizations that sponsor any type of mentoring process will gain. They also need to reach out to staff who have been "out-networked" but still come to work and operate on their own terms, which can pose a problem for others who are complying with unit or organizational policies. An empowered manager can offer a realistic plan to assist the individual to get back into the network; an individual who does not adhere to the plan would be terminated. Keeping employees who blatantly buck the system and get away with it is not tolerable. Organizations need to support their administrators in dealing with personnel problems. If these types of problems are dealt with, they are less likely to crop up again and will reinforce the importance of adhering to organizational policies. A mentoring culture that encourages nurses to grow should flourish in settings where nurses are respected and recognized for their good work.

Fabre (2005) suggests several techniques to assist in decreasing patient errors and nurse turnover in her book, *Smart Nursing: How to Create a Positive Work Environment That Empowers and Retains Nurses.* The author promotes six management practices to assist nurses in dealing with the chaos in health care:

- Respect
- Simplicity
- Flexibility
- Integrity
- Communication
- Professional culture

Each of these practices (except simplicity) is fostered by a mentoring culture and has been referred to in some manner already in this book. The concept of simplicity is something for nurses to review. All of us should try to think more simply when we organize our work to accomplish goals. Perhaps instead of developing lists of tasks for people we delegate to, we should empower them to fulfill the job in whatever way they think is best. And instead of worrying about being sure to create the perfect team or join the right network, we should realize that if we are open to encouraging others, the groups will form naturally (Wheatley, 2006).

Cleary and Rice (2005) look at collaboration between schools of nursing, state government, and health care institutions in strategizing ways to manage the nursing shortage. There are multiple initiatives that staff nurses need to be involved in so that the nursing workforce is developed most prudently. Katzenbach and Khan (2010) have a tool, *Assessing*

Your Organizational Quotient, to measure your organization's readiness to use both informal and formal lines of communication, which is available in their book, *Leading Outside the Lines: How to Mobilize the (In) formal Organization, Energize Your Team, and Get Better Results.*

IMPACT OF HAVING A MENTORING CULTURE FOR MENTORS AND MENTEES

The reason every nurse needs a mentor is that each nurse is different and a recipe or a one-size-fits-all mentality is not going to be effective. There is a greater need for mentoring models for preparing nurse leaders, developing a diverse nurse workforce, and preparing nurse scholars, if the profession of nursing wants to lead in the new health care reform.

Mentors in academia can guide a student with his or her research over one semester, connect the student to a funded researcher in the mentee's field, or advise by means of e-mail during a sabbatical and still have mentored or coached them. Many nurses connect with mentors over the Internet and communicate through e-mail. This is just another way of obtaining advice, and it is beneficial to have someone outside one's own institution or even one's field as one of the mentors in the multiple mentoring model (Whiting & de Janesz, 2004). The idea of the classic long-term dyad relationship is not the only type of mentoring there is, and more and more nurses will be accessing multiple mentors across their careers or engaging in group mentoring.

What about mentoring the more experienced nurse who, although does not want to live and work the "status quo," would like to gain more information or expertise or gain ways to keep what they have learned? This idea would reinforce the Master–Apprentice Model of tradesmen and women, where individuals work with others to maintain and gain skills and take on apprentices to teach and also to learn new techniques. Nakamura and Shernoff (2009) offer some good strategies for maintaining, as well as sharing, the present and past of a profession in their book *Good Mentoring: Fostering Excellent Practice in Higher Education.* Mentoring is a time-honored tradition and an important catalyst for people in achieving success in personal, professional, economic, and emotional areas.

For example, beginning staff nurses need seasoned, experienced preceptors to guide them through the maze of nursing in order to achieve the competency level. It will be more up to a peer mentoring network for nurses to proceed to the proficiency level and, for nurses who are very fortunate, the expert status. Benner's (Benner, 1984; Benner, Tanner, & Chesla, 2009) *Acquisition of Skills Model* is important for both mentors and mentees to review since it clearly identifies behaviors at each level of nursing expertise. It is only by having a standard by which to measure one's competency that the mentee can progress and accomplish his or her goals.

Mentoring is defined as any supportive relationship in which the individual or mentee receives guidance and encouragement. Often this guidance is reciprocal, that is, it is given back and forth between mentor and mentee. Peer or co-mentoring is a phenomenon that has caught on with the great majority of 20- and 30-year-olds. The guidance or coaching from peers can occur with a variety of learning opportunities: practicing and mastering clinical skills, tutoring for the National Council Licensure Examination (NCLEX) or a certification exam, offering strategies for succeeding with conflict management and departmental problems, offering troubleshooting advice for technology adjustments, obtaining federal funding for research, career planning, editing manuscripts, connecting individuals to networks, and legal or ethical advice, among many others. Other opportunities that mentors can help others with refer to providing experience to practice a specific skill—leadership, management, or clinical skills, for example. Mentors can also role model for mentees how to deal with particularly tough negotiations, policy development strategizing, and multiple challenging situations. Mentors also have a responsibility to instill pride in mentees and to role model for them that pride matters more than money (Katzenbach, 2000, 2003; Katzenbach & Khan, 2010).

CONCLUSION

Periodically, it is beneficial to review the various mentors one has or has had. Not everyone will have a legendary mentor. There is a tendency to have mentors when one makes a change in career or during shifts from one developmental stage to another in one's professional growth, but more and more, there is a high frequency of people always having a mentor via a multiple mentoring program. Hopefully, people can identify their mentors/preceptors/coaches/role models earlier in their careers and also use both informal and formal lines to make connections with larger mentor networks. But there are always some who are too arrogant to think they ever had a mentor and feel they achieved their career accomplishments solely by themselves. They do not realize the power of a team and often prefer to work in isolation. It is essential that these nurses realize what Kaplan and Norton (2004) emphasize: "No asset has greater potential for an organization than the collective knowledge possessed by all of its employees" (p. 63), and in order to make change in a macrosystem such as a health care institution one will need to be a member of a team or teams. So, individuals need to see if they can stretch some themselves by being more flexible regarding an idea or issue before they can attempt to change their organization. "Change something about yourself before trying to change something about your organization" is a good mantra to pilot one's career and even experience each workday (Katzenbach & Khan, 2010, p. 195). More change can happen in a work environment if one is in a mentoring culture atmosphere where there is dynamic exchange of ideas. Also, nurses need to remember that new graduates do tend to change jobs after the first and third year of beginning work as a staff nurse, but we can all support the concept of job embeddedness and try to inculcate a strong mentoring culture for nurses to have more reasons to stay than leave.

Most frequently, a mentor empowers an individual in some unique way to accomplish goals. Having self-esteem will allow the mentee to recognize others for their assistance. It seems that the more mentors one has, the more of one's potential is actualized, and the more accomplishments one experiences. It is probably correct to assume that the number of positive mentoring encounters far exceeds the small number of negative ones. How fortunate for those who can visualize having had a mentoring connection that included encouragement, challenges, constructive feedback, role modeling, and, for the mentor "to [be able to] fall back willingly to allow the mentee to walk beyond" (Schwiebert, 2000, p. 169). Even being able to give one or two of these gifts to another will facilitate the mentoring culture in nursing. If the mentoring culture is to take root, it is important that every individual, not just the academics, strive to fulfill more global goals in order to benefit the profession.

REFERENCES

Benner, P. (1984). *From novice to expert: Excellence and power in clinical nursing practice.* Menlo Park, CA: Addison-Wesley.

Benner, P., Tanner, C., & Chesla, C. (2009). *Expertise in nursing practice: Caring, clinical judgment, and ethics* (2nd ed.). New York, NY: Springer.

Bennis, W. (2003). *On becoming a leader: Leadership classic—updated and expanded* (2nd ed.). Reading, MA: Addison-Wesley.

Chitty, K. K., & Black, B. P. (2011). *Professional nursing: Concepts and challenges* (6th ed.). St. Louis, MO: Elsevier Saunders.

Cleary, B., & Rice, R. (Eds.). (2005). *Nursing workforce development: Strategic state initiatives.* New York, NY: Springer.

Fabre, J. (2005). *Smart nursing: How to create a positive work environment that empowers and retains nurses.* New York, NY: Springer.

Gilmore, J. A., Kopeikin, A., & Douche, J. (2007). Student nurses as peer mentors: Collegiality in practice. *Nurse Education in Practice, 7*(1), 36–43.

Halfer, D. (2007). A magnetic strategy for new graduate nurses. *Nursing Economic$, 25*(1), 6–12.

Halfer, D. (2011). Job embeddedness factors and retention of nurses with one to three years of experience. *The Journal of Continuing Education in Nursing, 42*(10), 468–476.

Halfer, D. & Graf, E. (2006). Graduate nurse perceptions of the work experience. *Nursing Economic$, 24*(4), 150–155.

Halfer, D., Graf, E., & Sullivan, C. (2008). The organizational impact of a new graduate pediatric nurse mentoring program: Background and significance. *Nursing Economic$, 26*(4), 243–249.

Heifetz, R. A., Grashow, A., & Linsky, M. (2009). *The practice of adaptive leadership: Tools and tactics for changing your organization and the world.* Boston, MA: Harvard Business Press.

Jakubik, L. D. (2008). Mentoring beyond the first year: Predictors of mentoring benefits for pediatric staff nurse protégés. *Journal of Pediatric Nursing, 23*(4), 269–281.

Jakubik, L. D., Ellades, A. B., & Gavriloff, C. L. (2012). Nurse mentoring study demonstrates a magnetic work environment: Predictors of mentoring among pediatric nurses. *Journal of Pediatric Nursing, 26*(2), 156–164.

Jokelainen, M., Turunen, H., Tossavainen, K., Jamookeeah, D., & Coco, K. (2011). A systematic review of mentoring nursing students in clinical placements. *Journal of Clinical Nursing, 20*(19/20), 2854–2867.

Kaplan, R., & Norton, D. (2004). Measuring the strategic readiness of intangible assets. *Harvard Business Review, 82*, 52–63, 121.

Katzenbach, J. R. (2000). *Peak performance: Aligning the hearts and minds of your employees.* Boston, MA: Harvard Business School Press.

Katzenbach, J. R. (2003). *Why pride matters more than money: The power of the world's greatest motivational force.* New York, NY: Crown.

Katzenbach, J. R., & Khan, Z. (2010). *Leading outside the lines: How to mobilize the (in)formal organization, energize your team, and get better results.* San Francisco, CA: Jossey-Bass.

Kiefer, C. F., & Schlesinger, L. A. (2010). *Action trumps everything: Creating what you want in an uncertain world.* Duxbury, MA: Black Ink Press.

Meister, J. C., & Willyerd, K. (2010). *The 2020 workplace.* New York, NY: Harper Collins.

Metcalfe, S. E. (2010). Educational innovation: Collaborative mentoring for future nursing leaders. *Creative Nursing, 16*(4), 167–170.

Mitchell, T. R., Holtman, B. C., Lee, T. W., Sablynski, C., & Erez, M. (2001). Why people stay: Using job embeddedness to predict voluntary turnover. *Academy of Management Journal, 44*, 1102–1121.

Nakamura, J., & Shernoff, D. (2009). *Good mentoring: Fostering excellent practice in higher education.* San Francisco, CA: Jossey-Bass.

Park, M., & Jones, C. (2010). A retention strategy for newly graduated nurses: An integrative review of orientation programs. *Journal for Nurses in Staff Development, 26,* 142–149.

Ponti, M. (2009). Transition from leadership development to succession management. *Nursing Administration Quarterly, 33*(2), 125–141.

Satterly, F. (2003). *Where have all the nurses gone?* Amherst, NY: Prometheus.

Schwiebert, V. (2000). *Mentoring: Creating connected, empowered relationships.* Alexandria, VA: American Counseling Association.

Spain, K. M., Clements, P. T., DeRanieri, J. T., & Holt, K. (2012). When disaster happens: Emergency preparedness for nurse practitioners. *Journal of Nurse Practitioners, 8*(1), 38–44.

Wheatley, M. (2006). *Leadership and the new science: Discovering order in a chaotic world* (3rd ed.). San Francisco, CA: Berrett-Koehler.

Whiting, V., & de Janesz, S. (2004). Mentoring in the 21st century: Using the Internet to build skills and networks. *Journal of Management Education, 28,* 275–294.

Zachary, L. (2005). *Creating a mentoring culture: The organization's guide.* San Francisco, CA: Jossey-Bass.

Zachary, L. (2009). *Group mentoring.* Retrieved from http://humanresources.about.com/od/coachingmentoring/a/group_mentoring.htm

Annotated Bibliography

Allen, T. D., & Eby, L. T. (Eds.). (2007). *The Blackwell handbook of mentoring: A multiple perspectives approach*. Malden, MA: Blackwell.

This book is the source for theoretical approaches to studying the concept of mentoring as well as various research methods that have or could be integrated into studies regarding mentoring. It has a multidisciplinary perspective, which is eye opening to those of us in health care. These scholars of mentoring look at mentorships for youth, the community, students and faculty, and the employee and employer. They explain some creative multiple mentoring models that could be applied to nurses in many of the health care delivery settings where we work.

Also, the book describes multiple ways of describing the term *mentoring*, and some of the descriptions are quite unique. Some other areas that are discussed, and in a most interesting fashion, include diverse mentors and mentees, naturally occurring mentoring, and various aspects of the formal versus informal pairing of mentor and mentee debate.

Bolman, L. G., & Deal, T. E. (2011). *Leading with soul: An uncommon journey of spirit* (3rd ed.). San Francisco, CA: Jossey-Bass.

The authors depict "Steve's" journey in obtaining more than just the bottom-line, such as love, power, and significance. Examples of Steve's interactions with various people along his "journey" will allow the reader to rethink some of one's own experiences. Ideas as to how more than just the cost savings or revenue generation mantra will trigger new inspirations for one's work. This book describes the spiritual aspect of one's leadership and will inspire the mentor and mentee to gather more from their discussions of experiences. Mentors, coaches, and preceptors can role model this often not-seen aspect of leadership to their mentees and show that they too can truly make a difference with significant contributions to their work.

Daloz, L. A. (1999). *Mentor: Guiding the journey of adult learners*. San Francisco, CA: Jossey-Bass.

This book is extremely informative regarding the challenges of mentoring adults. Daloz believes that adults want to learn all that they can and to the best of their ability, or in other words, the adult learner is generally a motivated learner. Therefore, Daloz reinforces the very important role of the mentor who mentors adults, focusing on facilitating or guiding the mentee and not telling them what to do or doing for them. The adult mentee needs time to find what they want, time to experience the opportunities and the challenges that face them, and time to gain knowledge and expertise from these experiences. Many examples of how to best mentor adults are described in this book.

Ensher, E., & Murphy, S. (2005). *Power mentoring: How successful mentors and protégés get the most out of their relationships*. San Francisco, CA: Jossey-Bass.

Ensher and Murphy interview 50 of the most powerful leaders in various industries in the United States and share their stories and how mentoring relationships assisted them with their success. Many of these leaders say that their relationships with their mentors have been the major factor which propelled them to success. The authors point out that today we need to have multiple mentors and mentors from all different facets of our lives. Less and less people today stay in one organization and have a classic dyad mentor-protégé relationship.

This book is a good resource for people who develop mentoring models and programs and also if one is involved in training mentors to mentor. Additionally, the book is a must read for people who are in mentor–mentee relationships and want to improve them or for people who are contemplating beginning a mentorship.

Heifetz, R. A., Grashow, A., & Linsky, M. (2009). *The practice of adaptive leadership: Tools and tactics for changing your organization and the world*. Boston, MA: Harvard Business Review Press.

This book presents a new way of seeing leadership and "doing leadership" or leading in a changing world. The authors decided to call this adaptive leadership or leading adaptive change. This book offers multiple tools and tactics to assist people in seeing the possibilities—not a daydreaming but real progress. For example, in Chapter 21, Inspire People, the authors explain that everyone has the ability to acquire the skill to inspire. They are adamant that being inspirational is not just held by a few select charismatic people. They recommend ways by which the reader can increase their ability to inspire through practice. They are quick to point out, however, that it is significant that individuals develop their own distinct style of inspiring or "speaking from the heart." Since we are living in extraordinary times it means every individual must "find better ways to compete and collaborate" (p. 2). They advocate that the world "needs to build new ways of being and responding beyond the current repertoires of available know-how." (p. 2) This book follows the authors' *Leadership Without Easy Answers* and *Leadership on the Line* books, which you may want to read if the adaptive leadership framework is a framework you can see working for you in your organization.

Jackman, I. (Ed.). (2005). *The leader's mentor: Inspiration from the world's most effective leaders.* New York, NY: Random House.

'This book is a guide for living one's life and cultivating leadership skills or for leaders who want to review what makes a leader effective and how other leaders have succeeded. It is a compilation of multiple leaders' viewpoints regarding the leadership phenomenon and also how they believe one should lead. Jackman, the editor of this book, is quick to point out that it is difficult to describe or define leadership. Rather, there are many ways of describing leadership and ways to go about gaining more leadership skills. There are specific short narratives on several leaders such as Vince Lombardi, George Patton, Dwight Eisenhower, Martin Luther King, Jr., Gandhi, Rosa Parks, women CEOs, and Winston Churchill. A comprehensive bibliography on leadership books is also included.

Katzenbach, J. R., & Khan, Z. (2010). *Leading outside the lines: How to mobilize the (in)formal organization, energize your team, and get better results.* San Francisco, CA: Jossey-Bass.

Katzenbach and Khan (2010) recommend using both the formal approach of communication that consist of strategy, structures, processes and procedures, programs, initiatives, performance goals and metrics along with the informal elements of an organization's communication system. They call these informal intricacies of the organization's culture the "magic of the informal" and include shared values, informal networks, communities, and pride. They also say the informal networks are generally fueled by peers and not the upper echelon of the organization. In fact, the upper management may be totally unaware of these networks. The book blends the informal and formal lines and describes how work gets done in all types of organizations. There is also a helpful diagnostic tool, *Assessing Your Organizational Quotient*, that could be most helpful to any organization interested in knowing the difference between what one thinks is happening in an organization versus what is actually happening.

Linley, P. A., Harrington, S., & Garcea, N. (Eds.). (2010). *Oxford handbook of positive psychology and work.* New York, NY: Oxford University Press.

Composed of six parts, this text includes information on positive psychology and the changing world of work, positive organizational leadership, positive work environments for individuals and organizations, enabling a positive working life, models for positive organization, and looking to the future: challenges and opportunities. The overlying theme, which is spelled out in the above six parts, is shifting our thinking from being more of a pessimist and thinking "What is wrong?" to more of an optimist and thinking "What is right?" As the editors so aptly say: "Positive psychology gives us a framework for approaching organizational issues that is focused on discovering the best of what is and creating the conditions that will enable that 'best' to flourish." The book reinforces the importance of looking at people's inherent potential for development, what their own ideas are, if they want to actually make a difference, and that if the correct alignment of the people and the goals of the organization occur then the future will hold great promise.

Murray, M. (2001). *Beyond the myths and magic of mentoring: How to facilitate an effective mentoring process.* San Francisco, CA: Jossey-Bass.

This is a great book of resources to assist in developing a mentoring program of any type. There are checklists and step-by-step models to adapt your own ideas to and then create a mentoring model for your organization or individual needs. She also has some good ideas on how to assign mentors to mentees and vice versa. She takes into consideration multiple factors and then makes suggestions as to what type of mentorship would work for various types of needs. The book has some easy-to-read ideas that are helpful in considering even before one starts creating a mentoring model. Additionally, she gives some helpful suggestions in evaluating the program for the mentees.

Robinson, K. (2009). *The element: How finding your passion changes everything.* New York, NY: The Penguin Group (Viking).

The Element is a great book to read at once, in parts, or even again and again. It continues to inspire most readers to seek one's own goals and follow one's vision. When you need to think about what you have decided to be your work and personal paths or trajectories and have a stumbling block occur, it is great to be able to re-read this book. The way the author goes about helping the reader achieve the soul-searching everyone should do to obtain their highest dreams is definitely unique and worth reading. The author, Ken Robinson, shares short stories about multiple people who have accomplished their dreams and more. Included in the book are Paul McCartney, Gillian Lynne, international choreographer, Matt Groening, creator of *The Simpsons*, Richard Feynman, famous physicist, and Arianna Huffington, an acclaimed journalist. The stories reflect on the individuals' pasts and how they created their futures by pursuing their passions and not taking any of their strengths for granted. It would behoove any mentor or mentee to read this book.

Sinetar, M. (1998). *The mentor's spirit: Life lessons on leadership and the art of encouragement.* New York, NY: St. Martin's Press.

Sinetar uses the art of encouragement framework to explain the various intricacies of mentoring. She describes many ideas to assist one in mentoring others through her 12 lessons of mentoring, and also gives some suggestions for mentees. Each of her lessons is clearly described and suggests easy step-by-step directions to follow for implementation. The author makes it difficult for the reader not to want to mentor someone or others. She has two other books which are helpful to read and also gives good ideas to help one mentor another: *Do What You Love ... The Money Will Follow* and *To Build the Life You Want, Create the Work You Love: The Spiritual Dimension of Entrepreneuring.* Sinetar gives great rationales of why it is always best to work with others and not in a silo.

Stoddard, D. A., & Tamsay, R. (2003). *The heart of mentoring: Ten proven principles for developing people to their fullest potential.* Colorado Springs, CO: NavPress.

These authors are very thought provoking with their descriptions of how to develop people to their maximum potentials through various types of mentoring. They speak to developing both the mentee as well as the mentor. Also, they discuss in detail the benefits of the reverse mentoring for the mentor. It is a very easy read and flows smoothly and quickly. There is a great amount of information and the reader can learn, in my opinion, how to be an excellent mentor by reading this book. Of course, it would be great to have a mentor that one can role model, but if that is not available the authors share enough information and examples of effective mentoring that one could certainly create an extremely effective mentoring relationship.

Sullivan, C. G. (2004). *How to mentor in the midst of change* (2nd ed.). Alexandria, VA: Association for Supervision and Curriculum Development.

This book illustrates many ideas and strategies to improve one's mentoring ability. The main premise of the book is that mentors must have vision, be able to empower others to have positive self-esteem, and to facilitate the mentees to progress along their own vision while simultaneously developing their own mentoring skills to assist in mentoring others. The author suggests that each and every person, mentor, mentee, want-to-be, and maybes can benefit from gaining increased mentoring skills. She points out multiple trends that will impact us in America, among which two have great impact on the mentoring: (1) The United States will become a nation of minorities and (2) The old will far outnumber the young (p. 10). Both of these demographic findings will impact the future of nursing. She further reinforces the importance of mentors and mentees not having too narrow of a network, but rather, that all must reach out to different kinds of people to gain the most in creating new ideas.

Zachary, L. (2005). *Creating a mentoring culture: The organization's guide.* San Francisco, CA: Jossey-Bass.

This book is a most comprehensive collection of ideas and step-by-step instructions on how to develop a mentoring culture in organizations. The author focuses on the individual, the dynamics of the workplace, accountability, responsibility for one's work and welfare of the whole, and on the fact that life is not just working and being. The author shares a *Mentoring Culture Audit* tool that would be helpful to any organization considering creating a mentoring culture, or for a workplace that has one and wishes to obtain some feedback data. There are multiple exercises and checklists that would facilitate the develpment of a comprehensive mentorship and mentoring culture.

Zachary, L. J. (2009). *The mentee's guide: Making mentoring work for you.* San Francisco, CA: Jossey-Bass.

Various definitions of the mentoring process, the roles of mentor and mentee, the stages of the mentoring process, mentoring as a relationship, and the benefits of the mentoring relationship are discussed. The book is specifically a guide for the mentee. Just about every aspect of mentoring and how it impacts the mentee is covered, including how important it is for individuals to consider being a mentee and a mentor for others at any time in their life for personal reasons. The book emphasize that the mentoring process is not just for education, the work place, or for improving one's career. Everyone should have a mentor or role model who is there to listen and encourage.

The book has some great exercises in Chapter 7 such as making the transition from mentee to mentor, the mentoring motivation checklist, reflections on your experience as a mentee, the *Listening Dynamic Profile*, and a feedback checklist for mentors. Zachary also provides an excellent website on mentoring at http://humanresources.about.com/od/coachingmentoring/a/group_mentoring.htm.

Index